I0439507

The Everyday Mom's Guide to Being

Fit and *Fabulous*

By: Shondreka Palmer

©2014 by Shondreka Palmer

ISBN 978-1499152296

All rights reserved. No part of this book may be reproduced, stored in a retrieval system, or transmitted in any form, or by any means, electronic, mechanical, photocopying, recording or otherwise, without prior permission of the author.

www.facebook.com/authorshondrekapalmer

www.twitter.com/authorpalmer

CONTENTS

Taking the First Step

Hello! Hello! Hello! I'm Shondreka and I'm a fit and fabulous mom! And so are you! In this book, I share my secrets and tips that have worked for me and helped me succeed in my weight loss journey. It took a lot of motivation, dedication, determination and hard work. But I did it - and so can you!

Disclaimer: Before starting any new diet and exercise program, please check with your doctor and get clearance for any exercise and/or diet changes. I am not a doctor or registered dietician. Any health, diet, or exercise advice is not intended as a medical diagnosis or treatment. Exercise at your own risk. The author and distributors of this book do not assume any liability for injury or loss in connection with this exercise program and instructions. This book is intended to share my story and hopefully inspire you on your journey to being a fit and fabulous mom!

Being fit and in shape is not all about being skinny, it's about being healthy - heart healthy. Living a healthy lifestyle that includes regular exercise and sensible eating habits can help protect you from heart disease, stroke, high blood pressure, diabetes, obesity, back pain, and osteoporosis. Regular exercise can also help improve and maintain your mood and it's an excellent way to help manage the stress in your life. A regular exercise routine may also be helpful in reducing feelings of depression and anxiety. Safety is always first when starting any new exercise regimen. You should always start out slowly and gradually increase your routine.

When you look good, you feel good! Why not take the first step and decide today to change your lifestyle and get started on a path that leads you to a healthier, fit you!

Good luck on your journey! I wish you great success!

Chapter 1

Just Me

I wanted to share a little history about me and my journey. For most of my life I've been physically fit and active. I didn't know how to be anything else. Well, at 25 years old my life changed forever. At that age, I found out that I was pregnant with my first child. Of course, I was overjoyed!! Who wouldn't be?! I'd heard the horror stories from other women that once you have a baby you can kiss your figure goodbye and that you would never look the same again. Years before I had my child, a family member told me, "You're all that now but wait until you have a baby". I thought to myself like most do-she doesn't know what she's talking about. Well, from my pregnancy experience I was half right!

Knowing that I was pregnant, I expected to gain weight. Realistically you have to gain some weight in order to support the new human being developing inside of you. I expected to gain about 30 pounds or so. And like I'm sure we all think, I thought *it's only baby weight, it will all fall off once I deliver my baby right?*- Wrong! Completely wrong! In reality, I gained about 70 lbs. during my pregnancy. I'm still not sure how but I did. I ate fairly healthy throughout my pregnancy- no weird cravings or anything. I craved tomatoes and pickles, nothing abnormally high in calories. Now in hindsight, I can understand why I gained so much weight during pregnancy. Though I was not eating unhealthy high calorie foods I was eating all the time. I stayed active and continued walking throughout my pregnancy. But that wasn't enough because I was consuming more calories than I was putting out.

To my surprise, I only lost about 10-15 lbs. after delivery of my son. Most of that weight was my son; he was a 9 lb. baby (smiles, love him!). I came to the realization that the weight was there to stay. Along with the weight shocker, my body was a shocker to me too. Since I've always been toned and fit most of my life, I naturally expected to be exactly the same afterwards. Well, that wasn't the case. My skin after pregnancy was loose. All muscle definition in the thighs, legs, arms and stomach were gone. My six pack was gone. But I had this wonderful, beautiful, healthy baby boy and I was thrilled with him! My post-pregnancy body was not what I expected but I knew that I would be back to be me in the long run. And guess what? I did it and so can you! Let the journey begin…

Chapter 2

Let's Go Get It!

Losing weight is very simple. In order to lose weight you have to extract more calories than you consume. Piece of cake right? Well it looks simple in writing and it sounds simple when you say it; but the act of doing this is extremely hard. Being consistent with it is an even harder task. But fear not, you can do it. I have faith in you. I did it then and continue to do it. Here are the ingredients: Start with healthy eating habits, add a dose of sweat, mix a little bit of determination, dedication and commitment and there you go. You are now fit and fabulous. Let's go!

First things first- healthy eating habits are a must. In my experience you can work out as much as you want but if your lifestyle is not combined with healthier, sensible eating habits you will not lose weight. Dare I say it- you may even gain weight. Now you ask, how can I gain weight when I work out regularly? Remember the key to weight loss is putting out more calories daily than you consume by food intake. We eat to live- not live to eat!

A pound of body fat equates to 3500 calories. It takes a loss of 3500 calories to lose one pound. If you have a calorie deficit of 500 calories (meaning that you burn 500 more calories than you eat each day) you will lose about 1 pound per week. Your goal should be to lose about 1-2 pounds per week. This will ensure that you lose the weight in a healthy manner. It also ensures that once you meet your weight goal you will be more likely to maintain it and not gain the weight right back. I know losing 1-2 pounds per week doesn't sound like a lot, but realize that successful weight loss takes time and more importantly, it takes consistence. Think of it like this - you did not gain the weight overnight so you can't expect to lose the weight overnight. In my case, I gained my weight over a 10 month time period. When I set the goal to get completely back in shape, I knew realistically to expect it to take about 10 months or so to get back to my fit and fabulous body. Also, consider it this way - as you are losing body fat you want to allow your body the time it needs to regroup and build muscle. If you try to lose weight too quickly your body will not have the opportunity to build muscle tone and you run a higher risk of having loose, sagging skin. So take a deep breath, put on your determination hat and get started.

To begin, I am not a calorie counter. I just cannot do it and I am not interested in counting every calorie I consume. For me, doing so brings on unnecessary stress. Plus it makes you feel like you are on a diet. Personally, I do not like the word "diet". I'm all about living a healthy lifestyle which consists of regularly making healthier food choices. The key to healthy eating is having the sweet, sugary, high calorie foods and drinks (foods we would normally consider junk food) in moderation. For me, I may eat "junk food" in a moderate portion about once every few weeks. When I am craving something "sweet" I make it a healthy sweet choice -like fruit. Don't look at eating healthier as depriving yourself; view it from the perspective of the glass is half full and you are choosing a healthier you! And who wouldn't want that?!

Now let's talk cost. Yes, eating healthier is slightly more costly than eating "convenience foods". But look at it this way- eating healthier is cheaper than the medical cost associated with high blood pressure, diabetes, cholesterol, etc. When you look at it that way the slightly increased grocery bills are worth it. It's the best money I've spent!

As stated earlier, I'm not the "diet" type of girl. So, just to give you an idea of what healthy food choices are, here are a few of my favorite selections that I eat on a regular basis. As you can see, I'm not eating rice cakes all day!

Breakfast

Bagels

Honey Nut Cheerios® with 2% Milk

Homemade Pancakes

Homemade Strawberry Banana Smoothie

2 Hardboiled Eggs

3-4 Slices of Turkey Bacon

Grits

Oatmeal

Fresh Fruit

Waffles

2 Scrambled Eggs

Beef Sausage

<u>Lunch</u>

Chef Salad topped w/ Pineapples, Apples,
or Strawberries

Soup

Turkey Sandwich

Tuna w/ Crackers

Grilled Cheese

Homemade Strawberry Banana Smoothie

Chicken Quesadillas

Pasta Salad

Grilled Chicken Sandwich

Dinner

Black Bean Salad

Vegetables- corn, green peas, green beans, zucchini, etc.

Baked Chicken Breast

Grilled Chicken

Pasta Entrées

Black Beans

Spaghetti w/Light Sauce

Snacks

Apples w/Cheese

Apples w/ Vanilla Wafers or Graham Crackers

Strawberries, Peaches, Pineapples, Watermelon, etc.

Tomatoes and Pickles

Cucumbers

Apples w/ Caramel Dip

Carrots w/ Ranch Dressing

Cheese and Crackers

Celery and Peanut Butter

Drinks

Water

100% Juice

Keep in mind that this is just a small sampling of the healthy food variations I incorporate into my healthy eating lifestyle. There are other choices out there. You should generally eat 5-6 times a day, which would include your three main meals, breakfast, lunch and dinner along with 2-3 healthy snacks throughout the day.

The key to drinking smoothies is to make them at home to ensure they are in their healthiest form. You control what is put into your smoothie when you make it at home. Also keep in mind that, depending on the amount of fruit you use, smoothies are naturally sweet and need no additional sugar added. Always use 100% fruit juice when making your smoothie. Also, if I drink a smoothie for breakfast or lunch, I tend to count it as the main course of my meal (replaces breakfast or lunch). If you drink a full cup of smoothie and eat a full meal along with it, it can cause you to gain weight because you are consuming too many calories. Never eat a meal and drink a smoothie as your drink for the meal. A smoothie is a meal within itself.

The key to sticking to a healthy food regimen is to find healthy varieties of food choices and snacks that you like and make them right for you. The list I provided works for me and I'm able to stick with my healthy lifestyle because I like eating these foods. You may not like anything that I select - and that's ok. There are many options available, so try them and see what you like and don't like and go from there!

Chapter 3

Begin! Days 1 ~7

Though I do enjoy being fit and healthy; I'm like most everyday people. I am not a fan of spending hours upon hours in the gym every day. Honestly, I do not have the time for that. I am a mother and I also work full-time. On top of being a mom I am a single parent, so all of the responsibilities associated within the household fall on me. (If you haven't checked out my first book, please do so! It is titled "Independently Raising a Man-Thoughts from a Single Mother's

Perspective". It is a positive, energetic, upbeat inspirational book that provides support and advice on how to manage life as a single parent. It's available on www.amazon.com.) With everything that I have on my plate, being healthy is a priority to me so I make time for it and commit to it.

If your goal is to lose weight and change your body, it's best to consistently work out 5 days/week. Working out 3-4 days/week is ok and will keep you healthy and in shape, but it generally just helps you maintain your current weight. I work out consistently 5 days per week. My workout routine normally lasts about 35-50 minutes. I start off with 30 minutes of cardio and about 15-20 minutes of muscle strengthening exercises. When trying to tone your body and your stomach, cardio is the key ingredient. Doing thousands of sit-ups will not help you lose stomach fat and tone but regular cardio workouts will do so. The key to a successful workout routine and not reaching a plateau (occurs when you are working out but are not losing any weight or inches) is to always keep your body guessing. You never want to do the same exact workout routine day in and day out. And always keep a bottle of water close by. Keep yourself hydrated throughout your workout by drinking water frequently. If you need to take a break, take a quick break and jump right back into the workout. In this book, I will discuss my 60 day workout routine that has helped me jumpstart my healthy weight challenge and helps me keep those pounds off!

Before you begin your workout routine and healthy lifestyle journey, you want to know where you started from and how far you've come. You can accomplish this by measuring your body. Start by measuring your waist and measure your left thigh. Keep track of your numbers by writing them down in a journal, including the start date. Weigh yourself as well, just so you can track your progress from when you start to when you finish and reach your goals. To get the most accurate weight measurement, it is best to weigh yourself in the morning. Do not become obsessed with weighing yourself and get lost in the numbers. Sometimes your weight may change slowly but you are losing inches, essentially becoming healthier and changing your body. Weigh yourself and measure your waist and thigh once every two weeks and write the results down in your journal.

Stretching before you start any workout routine is very critical. Warming your muscles up before you begin any exercise is necessary to prevent muscle strain and injury. Be sure to stretch all of your muscles before starting. During my routine, I always keep in mind that working out should not be painful. You should feel the burn, but nothing else. Stop if any pain exists and consult your doctor.

I get bored easily, so I'm always switching up my routine. Some days I start by doing 15 minutes of walking on the treadmill, other days, I start off by doing 30 minutes on the treadmill. After completing my cardio workout three days out of the week, I include strengthening workouts at the end of my routine. I usually complete 3 strengthening exercises with a focus on a specific muscle group. Of course, I cannot work out without my music, so I always have it along with me - jamming! In my experience, I have found that working out with music versus watching TV keeps me more focused on my workout and makes it more enjoyable for me. Try out different variations and see what works best for you and keeps you motivated to finish! I know far too well that being a busy mom with loads of responsibility leaves very little time to commit to a long workout routine. This is why my workouts last anywhere from 35 to 50 minutes. As mothers, it's important for us to make an effort to find this amount of time to commit to taking care of ourselves and our health. After all, we all need our health to manage the stresses of life and keep up with our busy schedules - *BEGIN!!*

As stated earlier, the key to a successful workout regimen is to keep your body guessing and not doing the same exact workout, day in and day out. To have the most effective workout routine, it is crucial that you have workouts that include low intensity days and high intensity days. High intensity workouts include what I like to call *"Energy Shots"*. Energy Shots are small bursts of rapid activity added in your workout that last about 30-60 seconds. Another key component to putting your safety first and ensuring a successful workout is to never work out the same muscle groups back to back. Always ensure there is a day or two between working the same muscles groups. For example, if you work out your lower body muscles (legs and thighs) on Monday, you should not workout these muscles again until at least Wednesday. Allowing your muscles time to take a break ensures they get the adequate rest needed between work outs to begin the toning and definition process.

Day 1 - Lower Body

<u>Pre-Workout Stretch</u>

Begin your routine by stretching your legs, arms, and neck muscles. Hold each stretch for a minimum of 20-30 seconds. This includes your hamstrings, quadriceps, glutes, calves, shoulders, back, stomach, triceps, and biceps. Remember, stretching prior to working out helps prevent injury. Throughout your exercise, remember to breathe regularly. Take in deep breaths through your nose and release them out through your mouth. Commit to memory that we pull our inner strength from our core (stomach) so always keep your stomach muscles firm and tight throughout the length of your workout.

<u>Cardio</u>

Treadmill

- Walk 15 minutes
- Random Mode
- 2.5 mph
- Level 1

Elliptical

- 15 minutes in forward direction
- Level 1
- 3.0 mph

<u>Squats</u>

Squats are an excellent lower body workout that target strengthening and toning your legs and buttocks. To begin squats, plant your feet flat on the ground about shoulder width apart. Point your feet slightly outward. Never let your knees extend beyond your toes. Slowly bend your knees as if you are going to sit in a chair with your butt pointing out. Hold your stomach muscles tight. Keep your back straight. In a controlled manner, slowly lower your legs down in a sitting position while placing your buttocks down and back. Ensure your upper legs are nearly parallel with the floor. To return to the standing position, push up on your heels and slowly lift up while maintaining a good safe form. Complete 3 sets of 10. (See picture on next page).

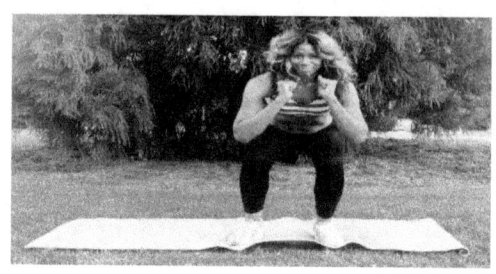

<u>Dead Lifts</u>

Start this exercise standing up in an upright position with your knees slightly bent and legs close together. Allow your arms to hang loosely and slowly come forward, bending at the waist. Keep your back straight and parallel to the ground as you are bending over towards your legs. As you complete the exercise, hold your stomach and butt muscles tight. Slowly come back up to a standing position. As you reach the top, be sure to seal the exercise by giving your butt muscles a firm, tight squeeze. Complete 3 sets of 10. (See picture below).

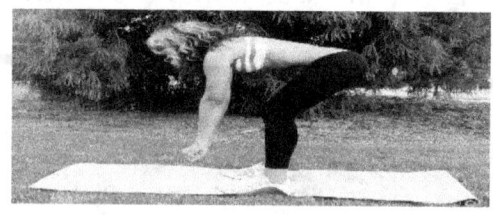

Front Knee Leg Lifts

While balancing on your right leg bring your left leg up slowly towards your chest. Extend your arms straight out to your sides. As you bring your leg up, be sure to hold it at a 90 degree angle. Pull your strength from your inner core and hold your stomach and butt muscles tight. Hold your leg up in the 90 degree angle for 5 seconds. Complete 3 sets of 10. Repeat with the other leg.

Cool Down Stretch

End your routine by stretching your legs, arms, and neck muscles. Hold each stretch for a minimum of 20-30 seconds. This includes your hamstrings, quadriceps, glutes, calves, shoulders, back, stomach, triceps and biceps. Take deep breaths in through your nose and out through your mouth. Stretching at the end of your workout is just as important as stretching before your workout. It important to bring your heart rate back down slowly and gradually.

Day 2 -Cardio Only

Pre-Workout Stretch

Begin your routine by stretching your legs, arms, and neck muscles. Hold each stretch for a minimum of 20-30 seconds. This includes your hamstrings, quadriceps, glutes, calves, shoulders, back, stomach, triceps, and biceps. Remember, stretching prior to working out helps prevent injury. Throughout your exercise, remember to breathe regularly. Take in deep breaths through your nose and release them out through your mouth. Commit to memory that we pull our inner strength from our core (stomach) so always keep your stomach muscles firm and tight throughout the length of your workout.

Cardio

Treadmill

- Walk 30 minutes
- Random Mode
- 2.5 mph
- Level 1

Cool Down Stretch

End your routine by stretching your legs, arms, and neck muscles. Hold each stretch for a minimum of 20-30 seconds. This includes your hamstrings, quadriceps, glutes, calves, shoulders, back, stomach, triceps and biceps. Take deep breaths in through your nose and out through your mouth.

Day 3 -Rest

Congratulations on completing the first 2 days of your journey to a new, fit, healthy lifestyle! Enjoy Day 3 by taking the day off from exercising. Allow your body and muscles to take a day of rest. Be sure to continue with making healthier, sensible food choices today. Enjoy!

Day 4 -Abs

Pre-Workout Stretch

Begin your routine by stretching your legs, arms, and neck muscles. Hold each stretch for a minimum of 20-30 seconds. This includes your hamstrings, quadriceps, glutes, calves, shoulders, back, stomach, triceps and biceps. Remember, stretching prior to working out helps prevent injury. Throughout your exercise, remember to breathe regularly.

Take deep breaths in through your nose and out through your mouth. Commit to memory that we pull our inner strength from our core (stomach) so always keep your stomach muscles firm and tight throughout the length of your workout.

<u>Cardio</u>

Treadmill

- Walk 15 minutes
- Random Mode
- 2.7 mph
- Level 2

Elliptical

- 15 minutes in forward direction
- Level 2
- 3.0 mph

<u>Push-Ups</u>

Assume a face down position on the floor with your feet together. Place your hands on the floor palms down, shoulder width apart. Curl your toes up toward your head. Pull your inner strength from your core and tighten your stomach and butt muscles. Raise yourself up using your arms. Allow your hands and the balls of your feet to support your weight. Make a straight line from your head to your heels. Lower your torso to the ground until your elbows form a 90 degree angle. Keep your elbows close to your body to add more resistance. Your head should be facing forward. Lower your torso as far to the ground as you can. Raise yourself up by attempting to push the ground away from you. Breathe out as you push. Continue to push yourself up until your arms are almost in a straight position. Do not lock your arms. Complete 3 sets of 5. (See pictures below).

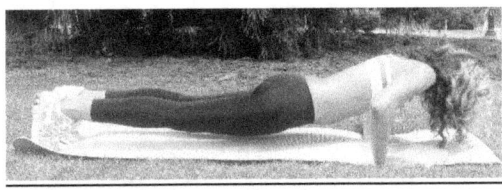

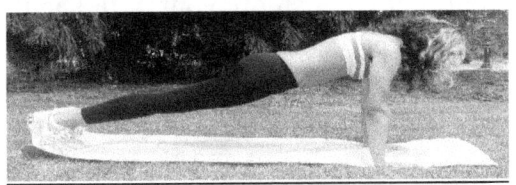

<u>Plank</u>

Start off in the push-up position with your hands placed on the floor palms down and shoulder width apart. Lower your forearms to the ground so that your elbows and fists are flat on the ground. Hold your abs and butt muscles tightly. Curl your toes under. Pull your belly button tight towards your spine. Your body should be positioned in a straight line. Keep your head down and your eyes on the floor in front of you. Hold this position for 30-60 seconds. Repeat 3 times. (See picture below).

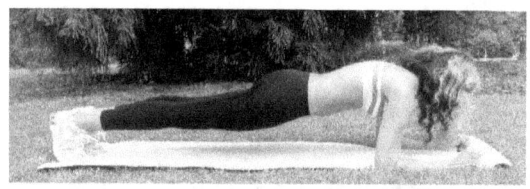

Side Plank

Start off by lying on the floor on your left side. Using your left elbow prop up the rest of your body. Position your left shoulder directly underneath your left elbow. Allow your right arm to rest on the right side of your body. Tighten your abdominal and butt muscles. Your body should be straight from your head to your feet. Do not allow your hip to sink in. Hold this position for 30-60 seconds. Complete 3 sets. Switch to your right side and complete 3 sets. (See picture on next page).

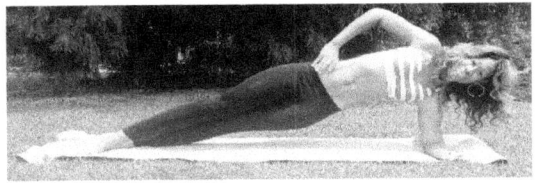

Cool Down Stretch

End your routine by stretching your legs, arms, and neck muscles. Hold each stretch for a minimum of 20-30 seconds. This includes your hamstrings, quadriceps, glutes, calves, shoulders, back, stomach, triceps and biceps. Take deep breaths in through your nose and out through your mouth.

Day 5 -Upper Body

Pre-Workout Stretch

Begin your routine by stretching your legs, arms, and neck muscles. Hold each stretch for a minimum of 20-30 seconds. This includes your hamstrings, quadriceps, glutes, calves, shoulders, back, stomach, triceps, and biceps. Remember, stretching prior to working out helps prevent injury. Throughout your exercise, remember to breathe regularly.

Take in deep breaths through your nose and release them out through your mouth. Commit to memory that we pull our inner strength from our core (stomach) so always keep your stomach muscles firm and tight throughout the length of your workout.

Cardio

Elliptical

- 30 minutes in forward direction
- Level 2
- 3.5 mph

Push-Ups

Assume a face down position on the floor with your feet together. Place your hands on the floor palms down, shoulder width apart. Curl your toes up toward your head. Pull your inner strength from your core and tighten your stomach and butt muscles. Raise yourself up using your arms. Allow your hands and the balls of your feet to support your weight. Make a straight line from your head to your heels. Lower your torso to the ground until your elbows form a 90 degree angle. Keep your elbows close to your body to add more resistance. Your head should be facing forward. Lower your torso as far to the ground as you can. Raise yourself up by attempting to push the ground away from you. Breathe out as you push. Continue to push yourself up until your arms are almost in a straight position. Do not lock your arms. Complete 3 sets of 5.

<u>Bicep Curls-No Weights</u>

Stand up straight with your feet shoulder width apart. Keep a slight bend in your knees while holding your stomach and butt muscles tight. Bend your right arm and hold it steady at a 90 degree angle. Keep your elbow in close to your ribs. With control, curl your right arm up to your shoulder. Lower your right arm back down to the start position. Complete 3 sets of 10. Repeat with the other side.

<u>Sky-Reacher</u>

Stand with your feet hip width apart. Step forward with your left leg, placing your weight on this leg. Lift your right leg up behind you. Bend forward slightly as you raise both arms over your head reaching up high. Hold your position for 30 seconds.

Repeat 6 times, alternating legs. (See picture below).

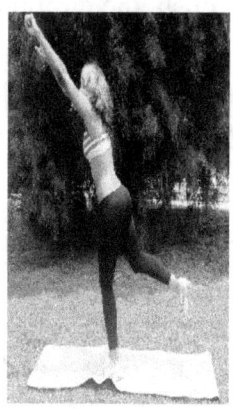

Cool Down Stretch

End your routine by stretching your legs, arms, and neck muscles. Hold each stretch for a minimum of 20-30 seconds. This includes your hamstrings, quadriceps, glutes, calves, shoulders, back, stomach, triceps and biceps. Take deep breaths in through your nose and out through your mouth.

Day 6 -Rest

You are doing a fantastic job so far and guess what?!? You are almost finished with the first week of your healthy, lifestyle journey.

Smile, give yourself a hand and pat yourself on the back! Today you will allow your body and muscles time to rest and take the day off from exercising. Enjoy it, but remember to eat healthy and sensibly throughout the day. Keep in mind that all the working out in the world will not keep your heart healthy or change your body if it is not paired with healthy, moderate eating habits. This is a lifestyle change! Keep going…you'll love the new, fit, healthier you when it's all said and done.

Day 7 -Cardio Only

<u>Pre-Workout Stretch</u>

Begin your routine by stretching your legs, arms, and neck muscles. Hold each stretch for a minimum of 20-30 seconds. This includes your hamstrings, quadriceps, glutes, calves, shoulders, back, stomach, triceps, and biceps. Remember, stretching prior to working out helps prevent injury. Throughout your exercise, remember to breathe regularly. Take in deep breaths through your nose and release them out through your mouth.

Cardio

Treadmill

- Walk 15 minutes
- Random Mode
- 2.7 mph
- Level 2

Elliptical

- 10 minutes in forward direction
- 5 minutes in reverse direction
- Level 2
- 3.5 mph

Cool Down Stretch

End your routine by stretching your legs, arms, and neck muscles. Hold each stretch for a minimum of 20-30 seconds. This includes your hamstrings, quadriceps, glutes, calves, shoulders, back, stomach, triceps and biceps. Take deep breaths in through your nose and out through your mouth.

Chapter 4

Week 2 Days 8-14

Awesome job completing your first full week of workouts! If you are not noticing a change in your weight, don't be alarmed. When starting a new workout routine it can take up to two weeks before you start seeing any changes on the scale. The scale should not be your main focus. As you continue your workout you will begin to see that you are losing inches and your clothes will begin to fit differently. This is assurance that you are making progress and are starting to make changes to your body. Remember, complete transformation takes consistency in exercising and eating a healthy, well-balanced diet. If you continue with your workouts and eating habits, you will see the weight come off over time. You will also begin to notice you feel healthier and more energized. Remember, fad diets change your weight but working out changes your body! Now let's move on the week 2!

Day 8 -Abs

<u>Pre-Workout Stretch</u>

Begin your routine by stretching your legs, arms, and neck muscles. Hold each stretch for a minimum of 20-30 seconds. This includes your hamstrings, quadriceps, glutes, calves, shoulders, back, stomach, triceps, and biceps. Remember, stretching prior to working out helps prevent injury. Throughout your exercise, remember to breathe regularly. Take in deep breaths through your nose and release them out through your mouth.

<u>Cardio</u>
Treadmill

- Walk 30 minutes
- Random Mode
- 2.8 mph
- Level 3

Bicycle Crunch

Begin this exercise by lying on your back. Place your hands behind your head. Raise your legs up bending them at a 90 degree angle. Pull your strength from your core and hold your stomach and butt mulches tight. Slowly lift your head up and bring your right elbow towards your left knee. Touch your elbow to your knee (the bicycle motion). At the same time, straighten out your right leg, ensuring it does not touch the ground. Switch sides. Touch your left elbow towards your right knee. At the same time, straighten out your left leg. Complete 3 sets of 10.

Sky-Reacher

Stand with your feet hip width apart. Step forward with your left leg placing your weight on this leg. Lift your right leg up behind you. Bend forward slightly as you raise both arms over your head reaching up high. Hold your position for 30 seconds. Repeat 6 times, alternating legs.

Ab Body Lift

Begin this position lying flat on your back with your arms and legs stretched out and fully extended. Pulling your strength from your inner core, hold your stomach and butt muscles tight. Slowly begin to lift your arms and legs at the same time off the ground slightly. Hold your head up. Hold the position for 30 seconds. Repeat 3 times. (See picture below).

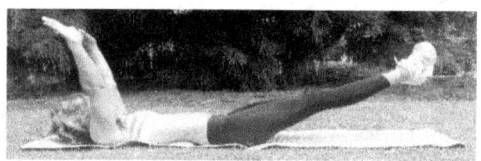

Cool Down Stretch

End your routine by stretching your legs, arms, and neck muscles. Hold each stretch for a minimum of 20-30 seconds. This includes your hamstrings, quadriceps, glutes, calves, shoulders, back, stomach, triceps and biceps. Take deep breaths in through your nose and out through your mouth.

Day 9 -Cardio Only

<u>Pre-Workout Stretch</u>

Begin your routine by stretching your legs, arms, and neck muscles. Hold each stretch for a minimum of 20-30 seconds. This includes your hamstrings, quadriceps, glutes, calves, shoulders, back, stomach, triceps, and biceps. Remember, stretching prior to working out helps prevent injury. Throughout your exercise, remember to breathe regularly. Take in deep breaths through your nose and release them out through your mouth.

<u>Cardio</u>

Elliptical

- 30 minutes in forward direction
- Level 2
- 4.0 mph

<u>Cool Down Stretch</u>

End your routine by stretching your legs, arms, and neck muscles. Hold each stretch for a minimum of 20-30 seconds. This includes your hamstrings, quadriceps, glutes, calves, shoulders, back, stomach, triceps and biceps.

Take deep breaths in through your nose and out through your mouth.

Day 10 Rest

Take the time today to relax and love yourself. You are off to a great start on your journey to achieving a new fit and healthier you! Keep your momentum up and your spirits high! By this time you should notice that you now have more energy. As busy moms, we all know that we need all the energy we can get to keep up with our active little ones and our agendas. Remember to eat healthy and sensibly throughout the day.

Day 11 - Upper Body

Pre-Workout Stretch

Begin your routine by stretching your legs, arms, and neck muscles. Hold each stretch for a minimum of 20-30 seconds. This includes your hamstrings, quadriceps, glutes, calves, shoulders, back, stomach, triceps, and biceps. Remember, stretching prior to working out helps prevent injury. Throughout your exercise, remember to breathe regularly. Take in deep breaths through your nose and release them out through your mouth.

Cardio

Treadmill

- Walk 30 minutes
- Random Mode
- 2.9 mph
- Level 3

Front Boxer Punches with Squats

Begin this position in a squat stance. Be sure your knees are positioned behind your toes. Bend your elbows so your fists are just below your chin. Pull your strength from your inner core and hold your stomach and butt muscles tight. Punch your right arm straight out. Pull it back in. Punch your left arm straight out. Pull it back. Start moving swiftly alternating both arms. Repeat for 30-60 seconds. Complete 3 sets.

Overhead Shoulder Press- No Weight

Begin this exercise standing in an upright position. Plant your feet firmly on the floor about hip width apart. Hold your arms straight out to the side at shoulder height. Pull your strength from your inner core and tighten your stomach and butt muscles. Bend your elbows at a 90 degree angle and slowly raise your upper arms up over your head in a controlled manner allowing your hands to briefly touch. Pull your arms back down to shoulder height, keeping your elbows bent at the 90 degree angle. Complete 3 sets of 12.

Standing Butterfly Press- No Weights

Begin this position standing upright. Hold your arms straight out to the sides. Bend your elbows up to a 90 degree angles with your palms facing outward. Hold your butt and ab muscles tight. In a controlled manner, bring your arms forward so that they meet in at the center of your chest. Pull your arms in together so that your elbows touch. Release and return to the starting position. Repeat. Complete 3 sets of 12. (See pictures on next page).

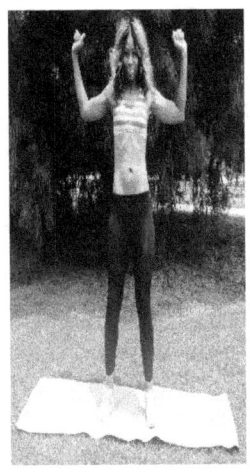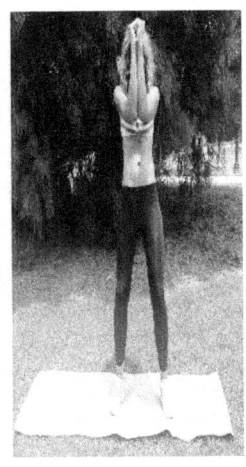

<u>Cool Down Stretch</u>

End your routine by stretching your legs, arms, and neck muscles. Hold each stretch for a minimum of 20-30 seconds. This includes your hamstrings, quadriceps, glutes, calves, shoulders, back, stomach, triceps and biceps. Take deep breaths in through your nose and out through your mouth.

Day 12 -Cardio Only

<u>Pre-Workout Stretch</u>

Begin your routine by stretching your legs, arms, and neck muscles. Hold each stretch for a minimum of 20-30 seconds. This includes your hamstrings, quadriceps, glutes, calves, shoulders, back, stomach, triceps, and biceps. Remember, stretching prior to working out helps prevent injury. Throughout your exercise, remember to breathe regularly. Take in deep breaths through your nose and release them out through your mouth.

Cardio

Elliptical

- 15 minutes in forward direction
- 15 minutes in backward direction
- Level 2
- 4.0 mph

Cool Down Stretch

End your routine by stretching your legs, arms, and neck muscles. Hold each stretch for a minimum of 20-30 seconds. This includes your hamstrings, quadriceps, glutes, calves, shoulders, back, stomach, triceps and biceps. Take deep breaths in through your nose and out through your mouth.

Day 13 - Rest

You've earned it! You are doing a superb job! Take the day off but remember to eat healthy and sensible throughout the day. Enjoy!

Day 14 - Lower Body

<u>Pre-Workout Stretch</u>

Begin your routine by stretching your legs, arms, and neck muscles. Hold each stretch for a minimum of 20-30 seconds. This includes your hamstrings, quadriceps, glutes, calves, shoulders, back, stomach, triceps and biceps. Remember, stretching prior to working out helps prevent injury. Throughout your exercise, remember to breathe regularly. Take deep breaths in through your nose and out through your mouth.

<u>Cardio</u>

Treadmill

- Walk 30 minutes
- Random Mode
- 2.9 mph
- Level 3

High Knees

Begin this exercise standing in an upright position with your feet placed about a hip width apart. Lift your right knee slightly higher than your hips pulling it up towards your chest. As you lower your right knee back down, start to bring your left knee up higher than your hip level. Continue to repeat by alternating your legs and lift them as high as you can. Move in a swift, quick manner.

As always remember to pull your strength from your inner core and hold your butt and ab muscles tight. Continue this exercise for 30-60 seconds. Repeat 3 times.

Butt Kicks

Butt kick exercises are completed while running in place. Position your body in an upright standing form. Your feet should be about shoulder width apart. Start jogging in place. As you are jogging in place ensure your butt and stomach muscles are engaged and tightened. While jogging in place bring your heels up to your glutes allowing them to touch your butt. Jog for 30-60 seconds. Repeat 3 times.

Butt Bridge w/ Leg Lifts

Start this position lying on your back with your knees bent and your feet flat on the floor. Place your hands underneath your head. Raise your hips so that your body forms a straight line from your shoulder to your knees. Pull your strength from your inner core and hold your butt and ab muscles tight. Slowly begin to lift your right leg straight out holding it at a 45 degree angle. Bring your right leg back in and place your foot back on the ground. Lift your left leg straight out holding it at a 45 degree angle. Bring your left leg back in and place your foot back on the ground. While lifting your legs up, ensure you keep your form and don't let your butt drop down. Continue this exercise alternating your leg lifts. Complete 3 sets of 10. (See pictures below).

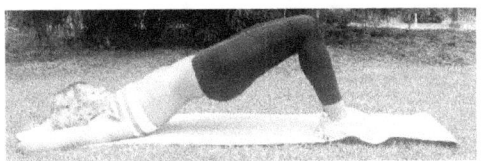

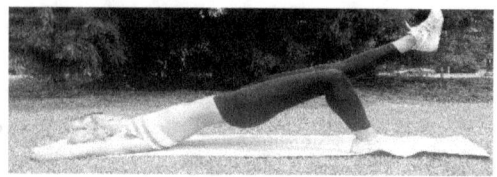

Cool Down Stretch

End your routine by stretching your legs, arms, and neck muscles. Hold each stretch for a minimum of 20-30 seconds. This includes your hamstrings, quadriceps, glutes, calves, shoulders, back, stomach, triceps and biceps. Take deep breaths in through your nose and out through your mouth.

Chapter 5

Week 3 Days 15-21

Well done! You've made it to week 3 of your healthy life challenge. I'm so proud of you and you should be proud of yourself too! Give yourself a hand and pat yourself on the back! You deserve it!

This week we will begin to maximize strength training by adding weights to the workouts. Adding weights will allow you to add more resistance. Strength training adds definition to your muscles and will aid in helping you sculpt your fit, toned body. It will also make you stronger as you get into better shape. On top of the physical attributes, strength weight training will also boost your energy level and improve your mood. This week we will be working out with 5 lb. dumbbell weights.

In addition to introducing weights to our program, we will also introduce speed intervals to our cardio workouts. Speed intervals are short bursts of vigorous activity. This is what I discussed earlier in the book and called them "*Energy Shots*". Energy Shots allow you to keep your body surprised and guessing and ensures your workout doesn't become stagnant; decreasing your chances of reaching a workout plateau (long periods of time in which you see no change in your body or weight loss). Weight training and speed intervals increase calorie burn both during and after exercise.

Do not be afraid to use weights during your workouts. There is a common false belief that women should not work out with weights because our bodies will bulk up and become too muscular like male bodies. This is completely untrue. Our bodies were not made to be as muscular as males. Unless you are getting additional hormone assistance from steroids, your body will not bulk up. When weights are used properly, they will tighten, tone, and sculpt your body. Enjoy your workouts this week. Remember to breathe, get your music out and most importantly have fun!

Day 15 - Upper Body

<u>Pre-Workout Stretch</u>

Begin your routine by stretching your legs, arms, and neck muscles. Hold each stretch for a minimum of 20-30 seconds. This includes your hamstrings, quadriceps, glutes, calves, shoulders, back, stomach, triceps, and biceps. Remember, stretching prior to working out helps prevent injury. Throughout your exercise, remember to breathe regularly. Take in deep breaths through your nose and release them out through your mouth.

<u>Cardio</u>

Elliptical

- 30 minutes in forward direction

- At 16 minute interval mark add an "Energy Shot". Increase your speed and pedal faster for 30-60 seconds. Resume normal speed.
- Level 3
- 4.5 mph

Bicep Curls-5 lb. Weights

Begin this position standing up with your feet hip width apart. Hold two 5 lb. dumbbell weights (one in each hand). Place your elbows in against your hip bone allowing your arms to slightly hang. Pull your inner strength from your core and hold your butt and ab muscles tight. Keeping your elbows firm at the hip bones, begin to lift both arms up until your forearm touches your chest. With control, move both arms back down to the starting position. Complete 3 sets of 10.

Butterfly Press- 5 lb. Weights

Begin this exercise standing up straight in an upright position. Align your legs so that they are hip width apart. Pull your strength from your core and hold your ab and butt muscles tight. Hold a 5 lb. dumbbell weight in each hand. Lift your arms up to shoulder height and bend them at a 90 degree angle. With control, move your arms inward toward your chest until the weights touch each other slightly. Move your arms back into the 90 degree angle starting position. Complete 3 sets of 10.

Push-Ups

Assume a facedown position on the floor with your feet together. Place your hands on the floor, palms down; shoulder width apart. Curl your toes up toward your head. Pull your inner strength from your core and tighten your stomach and butt muscles. Raise yourself up using your arms. Allow your hands and the balls of your feet to support your weight. Make a straight line from your head to your heels. Lower your torso to the ground until your elbows form a 90 degree angle. Keep your elbows close to your body to add more resistance. Your head should be facing forward. Lower your torso as far to the ground as you can. As your body gets stronger, you will be able to go lower. Start off slowly. Raise yourself up by attempting to push the ground away from you. Breathe out as you push. Continue to push yourself up until your arms are almost in a straight position. Do not lock your arms. Complete 3 sets of 6.

<u>Cool Down Stretch</u>

End your routine by stretching your legs, arms, and neck muscles. Hold each stretch for a minimum of 20-30 seconds. This includes your hamstrings, quadriceps, glutes, calves, shoulders, back, stomach, triceps and biceps. Take deep breaths in through your nose and out through your mouth.

Day 16 -Rest

You're now 3 weeks into your healthy lifestyle change. By this time, you should be feeling great! You should see an increase in your energy, along with your mood. Feel free to track your body progression by weighing yourself and measuring your stomach and left thigh. Track your results and write them down in your journal. Take the day off from exercising and enjoy yourself. Remember to eat healthy and sensibly throughout the day.

Day 17 -Cardio Only

<u>Pre-Workout Stretch</u>

Begin your routine by stretching your legs, arms, and neck muscles. Hold each stretch for a minimum of 20-30 seconds. This includes your hamstrings, quadriceps, glutes, calves, shoulders, back, stomach, triceps, and biceps. Remember, stretching prior to working out helps prevent injury. Throughout your exercise, remember to breathe regularly. Take in deep breaths through your nose and release them out through your mouth.

Cardio

Treadmill

- Walk 30 minutes
- At the 10 and 20 minute interval marks add an "Energy Shot". Increase your speed and jog faster for 30-60 seconds. Resume normal speed.
- Random Mode
- 3.0 mph
- Level 4

Cool Down Stretch

End your routine by stretching your legs, arms, and neck muscles. Hold each stretch for a minimum of 20-30 seconds. This includes your hamstrings, quadriceps, glutes, calves, shoulders, back, stomach, triceps and biceps.

Take deep breaths in through your nose and out through your mouth.

Day 18 - Lower Body

<u>Pre-Workout Stretch</u>

Begin your routine by stretching your legs, arms, and neck muscles. Hold each stretch for a minimum of 20-30 seconds. This includes your hamstrings, quadriceps, glutes, calves, shoulders, back, stomach, triceps, and biceps. Remember, stretching prior to working out helps prevent injury. Throughout your exercise, remember to breathe regularly. Take in deep breaths through your nose and release them out through your mouth.

<u>Cardio</u>

Elliptical

- 30 minutes in forward direction
- Level 3
- 4.6 mph

<u>Squats</u>

To begin squats, plant your feet flat on the ground about shoulder width apart. Point your feet slightly outward. Never let your knees extend beyond your toes. Slowly bend your knees as if you are going to sit in a chair with your butt pointing out. Hold your stomach muscles tight. Keep your back straight. In a controlled manner, lower your legs down into a sitting position while placing your buttocks down and back. Ensure your upper legs are nearly parallel with the floor. To return to the standing position, push up on your heels and slowly lift up while maintaining a good safe form. Complete 3 sets of 10.

Squat w/ Alternating Side Leg Lifts- 5lb. Weights

To begin this exercise, plant your feet flat on the ground about shoulder width apart. Hold 5 lb. weights, one in each hand. Hold your arms up, slightly bent. Keep your elbows in tight, pressing them against your sides. Point your feet slightly outward. Never let your knees extend beyond your toes. Bend your knees as if you are going to sit in a chair with your butt pointing out. Hold your stomach muscles tight. Keep your back straight. In a controlled manner, lower your legs down in a sitting position while placing your buttocks down and back. Ensure your upper legs are nearly parallel with the floor. To return to the standing position, push up on your heels and slowly lift up. Once you are back in the starting position, lift your right leg out to the side as high as you can. Bring your right leg back in. Complete another squat. This time when you return to the starting position, lift your left leg out to the side as high as you can. Continue completing a squat and then alternating the leg lifts. Complete 3 sets of 10.

Butt Bridge w/ Leg Lifts

Start this position lying on your back with your knees bent and your feet flat on the floor. Place your hands underneath your head. Raise your hips so that your body forms a straight line from your shoulder to your knees. Pull your strength from your inner core and hold your butt and ab muscles tight. Slowly begin to lift your right leg straight out holding it at a 45 degree angle. Bring your right leg back in and place your foot back on the ground. Lift your left leg straight out holding it at a 45 degree angle. Bring your left leg back in and place your foot back on the ground. While lifting your legs up, ensure you keep your form and don't let your butt drop down. Continue this exercise alternating your leg lifts. Complete 3 sets of 10.

<u>Cool Down Stretch</u>

End your routine by stretching your legs, arms, and neck muscles. Hold each stretch for a minimum of 20-30 seconds. This includes your hamstrings, quadriceps, glutes, calves, shoulders, back, stomach, triceps and biceps. Take deep breaths in through your nose and out through your mouth.

<u>*Day 19 - Cardio Only*</u>

<u>Pre-Workout Stretch</u>

Begin your routine by stretching your legs, arms, and neck muscles. Hold each stretch for a minimum of 20-30 seconds. This includes your hamstrings, quadriceps, glutes, calves, shoulders, back, stomach, triceps, and biceps. Remember, stretching prior to working out helps prevent injury. Throughout your exercise, remember to breathe regularly. Take in deep breaths through your nose and release them out through your mouth.

<u>Cardio</u>

Treadmill

- Walk 30 minutes
- At the 10 and 20 minute interval marks add an "Energy Shot". Increase your speed and jog faster for 30-60 seconds. Resume normal speed.
- Random Mode
- 3.0 mph
- Level 4

<u>Cool Down Stretch</u>

End your routine by stretching your legs, arms, and neck muscles. Hold each stretch for a minimum of 20-30 seconds. This includes your hamstrings, quadriceps, glutes, calves, shoulders, back, stomach, triceps and biceps. Take deep breaths in through your nose and out through your mouth.

Day 20~Rest

Another step closer! Take the day off from exercising and enjoy yourself. Remember to eat healthy and sensible throughout the day.

Day 21 -Abs

<u>Pre-Workout Stretch</u>

Begin your routine by stretching your legs, arms, and neck muscles. Hold each stretch for a minimum of 20-30 seconds. This includes your hamstrings, quadriceps, glutes, calves, shoulders, back, stomach, triceps, and biceps. Remember, stretching prior to working out helps prevent injury. Throughout your exercise, remember to breathe regularly. Take in deep breaths through your nose and release them out through your mouth.

<u>Cardio</u>

Elliptical

- 30 minutes in forward direction
- Level 3
- 4.7 mph

<u>Sky-Reacher- 5lb Weights</u>

Stand with your feet hip width apart. Holding a 5 lb. weight in each hand, step forward with your left leg placing your weight on this leg. Lift your right leg up behind you. Bend forward slightly as you raise both arms over your head reaching up high. Hold your position for 30 seconds. Repeat 8 times, alternating legs.

Plank

Start off in the push up position with your hands placed on the floor palms down and shoulder width apart. Lower your forearms to the ground so that your elbows and fists are flat to the ground. Hold your abs and butt muscles tightly. Curl your toes under. Pull your belly button tight towards your spine. Your body should be positioned in a straight line. Keep your head down and your eyes on the floor in front of you. Hold this position for 30-60 seconds. Repeat 3 times.

Bicycle Crunch

Begin this exercise by lying on your back. Place your hands behind your head. Raise your legs up bending them at a 90 degree angle. Pull your strength from your core and hold your stomach and butt mulches tight. Slowly lift your head up and bring your right elbow towards your left knee. Touch your elbow to your knee (the bicycle motion). At the same time, straighten out your right leg, ensuring it does not touch the ground. Switch sides. Touch your left elbow towards your right knee. At the same time, straighten out your left leg. Complete 3 sets of 10.

Cool Down Stretch

End your routine by stretching your legs, arms, and neck muscles. Hold each stretch for a minimum of 20-30 seconds. This includes your hamstrings, quadriceps, glutes, calves, shoulders, back, stomach, triceps and biceps. Take deep breaths in through your nose and out through your mouth.

Have Fun with It!!

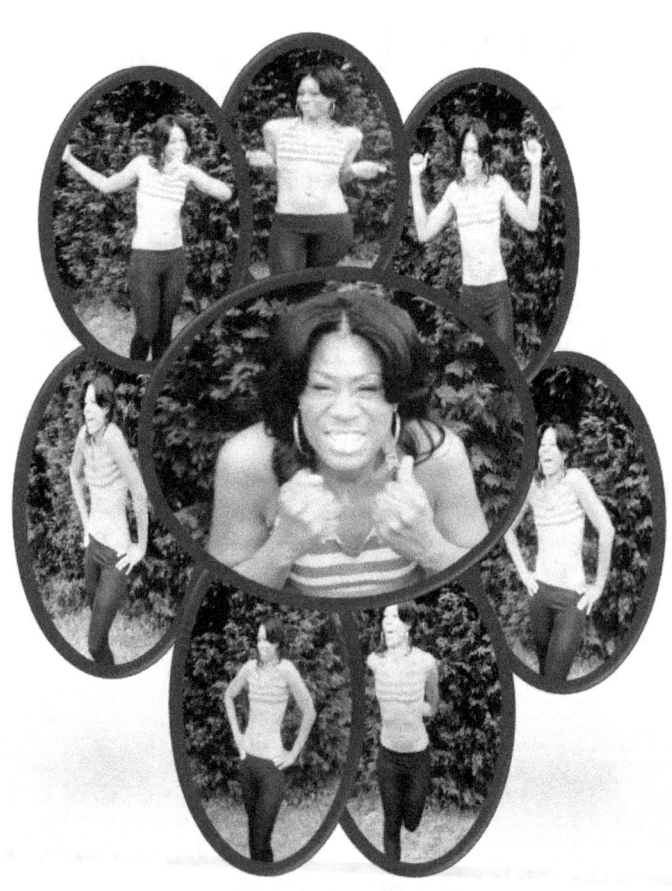

Chapter 6

Week 4 Days 22 -28

Yes! Feel pleased with yourself! You've made it to week 4 of your healthy life challenge. This week we will continue maximizing our strength training by working out with our 5 lb. dumbbell weights. We will also keep varying our workout intensity days by adding Energy Shots to our workout routine. Remember to keep it fun! Don't forget to breathe, and get your music out!

Day 22 - Lower Body

<u>Pre-Workout Stretch</u>

Begin your routine by stretching your legs, arms, and neck muscles. Hold each stretch for a minimum of 20-30 seconds. This includes your hamstrings, quadriceps, glutes, calves, shoulders, back, stomach, triceps, and biceps. Remember, stretching prior to working out helps prevent injury. Throughout your exercise, remember to breathe regularly. Take in deep breaths through your nose and release them out through your mouth.

<u>Cardio</u>

Treadmill

- Walk 30 minutes
- At the 10 and 20 minute interval marks add an "Energy Shot". Increase your speed and jog faster for 30-60 seconds. Resume normal speed.
- Random Mode
- 3.2 mph
- Level 4

Squats

To begin squats, plant your feet flat on the ground about shoulder width apart. Point your feet slightly outward. Never let your knees extend beyond your toes. Slowly bend your knees as if you are going to sit in a chair with your butt pointing out. Hold your stomach muscles tight. Keep your back straight. In a controlled manner, lower your legs down into a sitting position while placing your buttocks down and back. Ensure your upper legs are nearly parallel with the floor. To return to the standing position, push up on your heels and slowly lift up while maintaining a good safe form. Complete 3 sets of 10.

Standing Bicycle Kicks

Begin this position in a standing position with your legs positioned about hip width apart and your hands on your hip. Pull your inner strength from your core and hold your butt and ab muscles tight. Lift your right knee up to about hip height bending your knee at a 90 degree angle. Place your weight on your left leg. With control, begin to move your right leg in the manner you would if you were riding a bicycle. Kick your right leg out and then pull it back in to the 90 degree angle. Continue this motion. Complete 3 sets of 12. Repeat with the left leg.

Front Boxer Punches with Squat

Begin this position in a squat stance. Be sure your knees are positioned behind your toes. Bend your elbows so that your fists are just below your chin. Pull your strength from your inner core and hold your stomach and butt muscles tight. Punch your right arm straight out. Pull it back in. Punch your left arm straight out. Pull it back. Move swiftly, alternating both arms. Repeat for 30-60 seconds. Complete 3 sets.

Cool Down Stretch

End your routine by stretching your legs, arms, and neck muscles. Hold each stretch for a minimum of 20-30 seconds. This includes your hamstrings, quadriceps, glutes, calves, shoulders, back, stomach, triceps and biceps. Take deep breaths in through your nose and out through your mouth.

Day 23 - Cardio Only

<u>Pre-Workout Stretch</u>

Begin your routine by stretching your legs, arms, and neck muscles. Hold each stretch for a minimum of 20-30 seconds. This includes your hamstrings, quadriceps, glutes, calves, shoulders, back, stomach, triceps, and biceps. Remember, stretching prior to working out helps prevent injury. Throughout your exercise, remember to breathe regularly. Take in deep breaths through your nose and release them out through your mouth.

<u>Cardio</u>

Elliptical

- 30 minutes in forward direction
- At the 15 minute mark, pedal in reverse for 2 minutes; resume forward direction
- Level 3
- 4.8 mph

<u>Cool Down Stretch</u>

End your routine by stretching your legs, arms, and neck muscles. Hold each stretch for a minimum of 20-30 seconds. This includes your hamstrings, quadriceps, glutes, calves,

shoulders, back, stomach, triceps and biceps. Take deep breaths in through your nose and out through your mouth.

Day 24 -Rest

Wow! You are about a month into your new healthy, fit lifestyle! It feels great to be doing something for yourself, right? As moms, we get so caught up in taking care of everyone else that we forget how important it is to take care of ourselves. Enjoy your day of rest and remember to eat healthy and sensibly throughout the day.

Day 25 - Cardio Only

Pre-Workout Stretch

Begin your routine by stretching your legs, arms, and neck muscles. Hold each stretch for a minimum of 20-30 seconds. This includes your hamstrings, quadriceps, glutes, calves, shoulders, back, stomach, triceps, and biceps. Remember, stretching prior to working out helps prevent injury. Throughout your exercise, remember to breathe regularly.

Take in deep breaths through your nose and release them out through your mouth.

<u>Cardio</u>

Treadmill

- Walk 30 minutes
- At the 10 and 20 minute interval marks add an "Energy Shot". Increase your speed and jog faster for 30-60 seconds. Resume normal speed.
- Random Mode
- 3.2 mph
- Level 4

<u>Cool Down Stretch</u>

End your routine by stretching your legs, arms, and neck muscles. Hold each stretch for a minimum of 20-30 seconds. This includes your hamstrings, quadriceps, glutes, calves, shoulders, back, stomach, triceps and biceps. Take deep breaths in through your nose and out through your mouth.

<u>Day 26 - Abs</u>

<u>Pre-Workout Stretch</u>

Begin your routine by stretching your legs, arms, and neck muscles. Hold each stretch for a minimum of 20-30 seconds. This includes your hamstrings, quadriceps, glutes, calves, shoulders, back, stomach, triceps, and biceps. Remember, stretching prior to working out helps prevent injury. Throughout your exercise, remember to breathe regularly. Take in deep breaths through your nose and release them out through your mouth.

Cardio

Elliptical

- 30 minutes in forward direction
- At the 15 minute mark, pedal in reverse for 3 minutes; resume forward direction
- Level 3
- 4.8 mph

Planks

Begin this exercise in a push-up position. Slowly bend your arms and lower yourself down to the ground. Place your weight on your forearms. Your palms can either be flat to the ground or balled in a fist. Place your hands in the position that feels most comfortable to you. Your body should form a straight line. Curl your toes under and engage your stomach by tilting your pelvis and pulling your belly button toward your spine. Keep your eyes on the floor in front of you. Do not drop your hips or raise your butt. Hold this position for 30-60 seconds. Repeat 3 times.

Side Planks

Begin this exercise by lying flat on your left side with your legs straight. Use your left elbow to prop up the rest of your body. Ensure your body forms a diagonal line. Position your left elbow so that is directly underneath your left shoulder. Rest your right arm on your hip. Pull your strength from your inner core and hold your stomach and butt muscles tight. Your hips and knees should not touch the ground. Hold the position for 30-60 seconds. Repeat 3 times.

Butt Bridge

Start this position lying on your back with your knees bent and your feet flat on the floor. Rest your arms on the floor. Place your hands underneath your head. Raise your hips so that your body forms a straight line from your shoulder to your knees. Pull your strength from your inner core and hold your butt and ab muscles tight. Hold this position for 30-60 seconds. Repeat 3 times.

<u>Cool Down Stretch</u>

End your routine by stretching your legs, arms, and neck muscles. Hold each stretch for a minimum of 20-30 seconds. This includes your hamstrings, quadriceps, glutes, calves, shoulders, back, stomach, triceps and biceps. Take deep breaths in through your nose and out through your mouth.

Day 27 -Rest

Another successful day towards your healthy, fit lifestyle! Enjoy your day of rest and remember to eat healthy and sensibly throughout the day.

Day 28 -Upper Body

<u>Pre-Workout Stretch</u>

Begin your routine by stretching your legs, arms, and neck muscles. Hold each stretch for a minimum of 20-30 seconds. This includes your hamstrings, quadriceps, glutes, calves, shoulders, back, stomach, triceps, and biceps. Remember, stretching prior to working out helps prevent injury. Throughout your exercise, remember to breathe regularly. Take in deep breaths through your nose and release them out through your mouth.

Cardio

Treadmill

- Walk 30 minutes
- Random Mode
- 3.2 mph
- Level 4

Jumping Jacks

Start out standing up straight with your feet together and your arms at your sides. Bend your knees slightly and jump a few inches into the air. While in the air bring legs out to the side about shoulder width apart. As you move your legs outward, raise your arms up over your head. Be sure your arms are slightly bent throughout the movement. Your feet land shoulder width or wider as your hands meet above your head. Repeat this motion in a quick manner for 30-60 seconds. Repeat 3 times.

Bicep Curls- 5 lb. Weights

Stand in an upright position with your feet shoulder width apart. Hold 5 lb. dumbbell weights in each hand. Place your elbows against your hip bones, letting your arms slightly hang. Contract your stomach and butt muscles, holding them tight. Slowly lift both arms up together until your forearms reach your chest. Lift your arms back down to the starting position ensuring your elbows remain against your hip bones. Complete 3 sets of 15.

Shoulder Curls-5 lb. Weights

Stand in an upright position with your feet shoulder width apart. Hold 5 lb. dumbbell weights in each hand. Hold your butt and stomach muscles tight. Extend both arms out to the side, keeping them level with your shoulders. Palms should be facing up. Your elbows should be slightly bent. Begin to slowly curl your arms up toward your head, allowing your fists to slightly touch our shoulders. With control, begin to move your arms back outward, keeping your elbows slightly bent. Complete 3 sets of 15.

Cool Down Stretch

End your routine by stretching your legs, arms, and neck muscles. Hold each stretch for a minimum of 20-30 seconds. This includes your hamstrings, quadriceps, glutes, calves, shoulders, back, stomach, triceps and biceps. Take deep breaths in through your nose and out through your mouth.

Chapter 7

Week 5 Days 29-35

Y ou are now in week 5 of your healthy
lifestyle change. Don't you feel
incredible?!? You should definitely
start to see some changes in your mood and
body. Track your progress this week.
Measure your waistline, your left thigh and
weigh yourself. Write down the results in
your journal. We will continue maximizing
our strength training by working out with our
5 lb. dumbbell weights. We will also keep
varying our workout intensity days by adding
Energy Shots on most days of our workouts.

Remember to breathe, keep your water close by and have fun!

Day 29 Lower Body

<u>Pre-Workout Stretch</u>

Begin your routine by stretching your legs, arms, and neck muscles. Hold each stretch for a minimum of 20-30 seconds. This includes your hamstrings, quadriceps, glutes, calves, shoulders, back, stomach, triceps, and biceps. Remember, stretching prior to working out helps prevent injury. Throughout your exercise, remember to breathe regularly. Take in deep breaths through your nose and release them out through your mouth.

<u>Cardio</u>

Elliptical

- 30 minutes in forward direction
- At the 10 and 20 minute interval marks add an "Energy Shot". Increase your speed and pedal faster for 30-60 seconds. Resume normal speed.
- Level 4
- 4.9 mph

Standing Back Leg Lift

Stand up straight placing your hands on your hips. Slowly lift your right leg while balancing on your left foot. Bend your left knee slightly. Pull your inner strength from your core and tighten your ab and butt muscles. Extend your right leg back and out to a 45 degree angle. Balancing on your left foot, begin to lift your right leg up towards your butt. Give your butt a squeeze as you lift your leg. With control, bring your right leg back down to the starting position. Try not to let your right leg touch the ground. Complete 3 sets of 12. Switch to the other side and repeat. To start off, if you need help with your balance, you can use a chair to rest one hand on. As your endurance increases, you may not need the chair to support yourself while balancing.

Standing Side Leg Lifts

Stand up straight placing your hands on your hips. Slowly lift your right leg up slightly bending your knee while balancing your weight on your left foot. Bend your left knee slightly. Begin to extend your right leg out to your right side while balancing on your left leg. Lift your right leg out to about a 45 degree angle. With control, bring your right leg back down to the starting position. Try not to let your right leg touch the ground. Complete 3 sets of 10. Switch to the other side and repeat. If you need help with your balance you can use a chair to rest one hand on. (See pictures below).

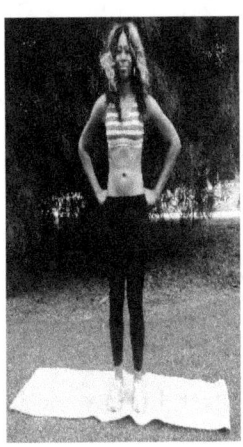 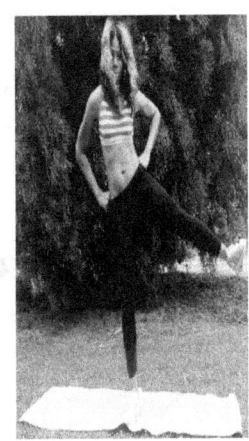

Butt Kicks

You will complete the butt kicks exercises while running in place. Position your body in an upright standing form. Your feet should be about shoulder width apart. Start jogging in place. As you are jogging in place ensure your butt and stomach muscles are engaged and tightened. While jogging in place bring your heels to your glutes allowing them to touch our butt. Jog for 30-60 seconds. Repeat 3 times.

Cool Down Stretch

End your routine by stretching your legs, arms, and neck muscles. Hold each stretch for a minimum of 20-30 seconds. This includes your hamstrings, quadriceps, glutes, calves, shoulders, back, stomach, triceps and biceps. Take deep breaths in through your nose and out through your mouth.

Day 30 -Cardio Only

Pre-Workout Stretch

Begin your routine by stretching your legs, arms, and neck muscles. Hold each stretch for a minimum of 20-30 seconds. This includes your hamstrings, quadriceps, glutes, calves, shoulders, back, stomach, triceps, and biceps. Remember, stretching prior to working out helps prevent injury. Throughout your exercise, remember to breathe regularly. Take in deep breaths through your nose and release them out through your mouth.

Cardio

Treadmill

- Walk 30 minutes
- Random Mode
- 3.3 mph
- Level 5

<u>Cool Down Stretch</u>

End your routine by stretching your legs, arms, and neck muscles. Hold each stretch for a minimum of 20-30 seconds. This includes your hamstrings, quadriceps, glutes, calves, shoulders, back, stomach, triceps and biceps. Take deep breaths in through your nose and out through your mouth.

<u>Day 31 -Rest</u>

Take a break from working out today. Remember to eat healthy and sensibly throughout the day. Don't forget fad diets change your weight but working out changes your body! Cheers to a healthy lifestyle!!

<u>Day 32 Abs</u>

Pre-Workout Stretch

Begin your routine by stretching your legs, arms, and neck muscles. Hold each stretch for a minimum of 20-30 seconds. This includes your hamstrings, quadriceps, glutes, calves, shoulders, back, stomach, triceps, and biceps. Remember, stretching prior to working out helps prevent injury. Throughout your exercise, remember to breathe regularly. Take in deep breaths through your nose and release them out through your mouth.

Cardio

Elliptical

- 30 minutes in forward direction
- At the 15 minute mark, pedal in reverse for 5 minutes; resume forward direction
- Level 4
- 4.9 mph

Plank with Arm Extension

Begin this exercise in the plank position. Ensure your toes and your forearms are on the floor. Pull your strength from your inner core and hold your butt and ab muscles tight. Your body should form a straight line. With control, shift your weight to your right forearm. Extend your left arm out in front of you and hold for 20-30 seconds. Slowly bring your arm back in. Repeat with the right arm. Complete 2 sets of 5.

<u>Ab Leg Lift</u>

Begin this position sitting up tall on the floor. Place your hands at your sides and extend your legs out in front of you. Pull your inner strength from your core and hold your ab and butt muscles tight. Lift your feet off the floor with your knees slightly bent and shins parallel to floor. With control, lean back slightly. Extend your arms straight out in front of you keeping them at shoulder height. Hold this position for 30-60 seconds. Repeat 3 times. (See picture below).

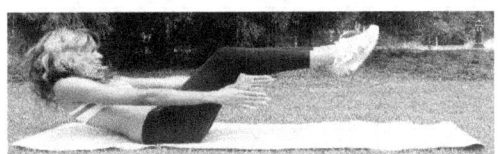

<u>Ab Roll Up</u>

Start this position lying on your back. Stretch your arms straight out behind you. Extend your legs so that you form a straight line. Pull your strength from your inner core and hold your ab and butt muscles tight. With control, lift your arms and upper body up off the floor. Roll your upper body and arms forward and touch toward your toes. With control, lower your upper body back down to the starting position. Complete 3 sets of 10.

Cool Down Stretch

End your routine by stretching your legs, arms, and neck muscles. Hold each stretch for a minimum of 20-30 seconds. This includes your hamstrings, quadriceps, glutes, calves, shoulders, back, stomach, triceps and biceps. Take deep breaths in through your nose and out through your mouth.

Day 33 - Cardio Only

Pre-Workout Stretch

Begin your routine by stretching your legs, arms, and neck muscles. Hold each stretch for a minimum of 20-30 seconds. This includes your hamstrings, quadriceps, glutes, calves, shoulders, back, stomach, triceps, and biceps. Remember, stretching prior to working out helps prevent injury. Throughout your exercise, remember to breathe regularly.

Take in deep breaths through your nose and release them out through your mouth.

<u>Cardio</u>

Treadmill

- Walk 30 minutes
- At the 10 and 20 minute interval marks add an "Energy Shot". Increase your speed and jog faster for 30-60 seconds. Resume normal speed.
- Random Mode
- 3.5 mph
- Level 5

<u>Cool Down Stretch</u>

End your routine by stretching your legs, arms, and neck muscles. Hold each stretch for a minimum of 20-30 seconds. This includes your hamstrings, quadriceps, glutes, calves, shoulders, back, stomach, triceps and biceps. Take deep breaths in through your nose and out through your mouth.

Day 34 -Rest

Oh yea! Another day down and another step in the right direction! Take a break from working out today and enjoy yourself! Remember to eat healthy and sensibly throughout the day.

Day 35 -Upper Body

Pre-Workout Stretch

Begin your routine by stretching your legs, arms, and neck muscles. Hold each stretch for a minimum of 20-30 seconds. This includes your hamstrings, quadriceps, glutes, calves, shoulders, back, stomach, triceps, and biceps. Remember, stretching prior to working out helps prevent injury. Throughout your exercise, remember to breathe regularly. Take in deep breaths through your nose and release them out through your mouth.

Cardio

Elliptical

- 30 minutes in forward direction

- Level 4
- 4.9 mph

Triceps Swing- 5lb Weights

Begin this exercise lying on your back with your knees bent and your feet flat on the floor. Spread your legs apart slightly about hip width apart. Hold 5 lb. dumbbell weights in each hand. Hold your arms straight back over your head. Pull your strength from your inner core and hold your stomach and butt muscles tight. While keeping your left arm straight, raise your right arm up over your chest. Lower your right arm back down to the starting position. Complete 3 sets of 12. Switch sides and repeat.

Opposite Arm & Leg Lift

Begin this exercise, lying on your stomach. Lift your body up on all fours. Your arms should be straight underneath your shoulders and you should be positioned on your knees. Pull your strength from your inner core and hold your stomach and butt muscles tight. Reach your right arm forward and at the same time stretch your left leg back. Hold this position for 10 seconds and then release. Repeat, this time using your left arm and right leg. Complete 12 reps.

Overhead Triceps Curls-5 lb. Weights

Begin this exercise by standing up straight. Spread your legs so that they are shoulder width apart. Hold a 5 lb. weight in each hand. Raise both arms up over your head, keeping your upper arms close to your head. Pull your strength from your inner core and hold your stomach and butt muscles tight. With control, lower your arms down; bending them at the elbows until your hands touch near the back of your shoulders. Return to the starting position. Complete 3 sets of 10.

Cool Down Stretch

End your routine by stretching your legs, arms, and neck muscles. Hold each stretch for a minimum of 20-30 seconds. This includes your hamstrings, quadriceps, glutes, calves, shoulders, back, stomach, triceps and biceps. Take deep breaths in through your nose and out through your mouth.

Chapter 8

Week 6 Days 36~42

Congratulations!! It's now week 6 of your healthy, lifestyle challenge! You are doing an awesome job!! Your body is stronger and it feels great, doesn't it?! Working out has so many benefits! As a busy mom, it can be easy to get stressed out. One of the greatest benefits of working out is it serves to manage stress. Be sure to continue to manage your life and schedule to always include time to yourself to work out. Working out does a body good! Now let's tackle week 6!

Day 36 -Abs

<u>Pre-Workout Stretch</u>

Begin your routine by stretching your legs, arms, and neck muscles. Hold each stretch for a minimum of 20-30 seconds. This includes your hamstrings, quadriceps, glutes, calves, shoulders, back, stomach, triceps, and biceps. Remember, stretching prior to working out helps prevent injury. Throughout your exercise, remember to breathe regularly. Take in deep breaths through your nose and release them out through your mouth.

<u>Cardio</u>

Treadmill

- Walk 30 minutes
- Random Mode
- 3.5 mph
- Level 5

<u>Leg Swing</u>

Start this exercise lying on your back. Hold your arms straight out at your sides with your palms face down or place your hands underneath your butt. Pull your strength from your inner core and hold your butt and ab muscles tight. With control, raise both legs up toward the ceiling. Your legs should be at a 90 degree angle to your hips. Slowly lower your legs down until they are about four inches above the floor (or as low as you can go without lifting the small of your back). Raise your legs back up to the starting position. Complete 3 sets of 4.

Scissor Kicks

Start this exercise lying on your back. Pull your strength from your inner core and hold your butt and ab muscles tight. Slowly raise both legs up toward the ceiling. Keeping them straight, lower your left leg until it's about six inches off the floor. Lift your head and shoulders off the floor and grab the back of your right leg, gently pulling it toward you. Switch legs and repeat on other side. Complete in a quick, swift manner, switching from leg to leg. Complete 3 sets of 10.

Reverse Plank

Begin this position sitting on the floor with your knees bent and your feet hip-width apart, flat on the floor. Place your palms on the floor on either side of your hips. Pull your strength from your inner core and hold your ab and butt muscles tight. Lift your butt off the floor until it is level with your hips and your torso is parallel to the floor. Holding this "table top" position for 30-60 seconds. Repeat 3 times. (See picture below).

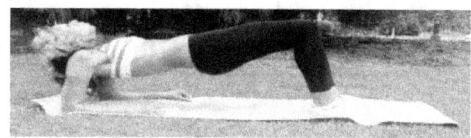

Cool Down Stretch

End your routine by stretching your legs, arms, and neck muscles. Hold each stretch for a minimum of 20-30 seconds. This includes your hamstrings, quadriceps, glutes, calves, shoulders, back, stomach, triceps and biceps. Take deep breaths in through your nose and out through your mouth.

Day 37-Cardio Only

Pre-Workout Stretch

Begin your routine by stretching your legs, arms, and neck muscles. Hold each stretch for a minimum of 20-30 seconds. This includes your hamstrings, quadriceps, glutes, calves, shoulders, back, stomach, triceps, and biceps.

Remember, stretching prior to working out helps prevent injury. Throughout your exercise, remember to breathe regularly. Take in deep breaths through your nose and release them out through your mouth.

Cardio

Elliptical

- 30 minutes in forward direction
- At the 10 and 20 minute interval marks add an "Energy Shot". Increase your speed and pedal faster for 30-60 seconds in reverse direction. Resume normal speed and return to forward direction
- Level 4
- 4.9 mph

Cool Down Stretch

End your routine by stretching your legs, arms, and neck muscles. Hold each stretch for a minimum of 20-30 seconds. This includes your hamstrings, quadriceps, glutes, calves, shoulders, back, stomach, triceps and biceps. Take deep breaths in through your nose and out through your mouth.

Day 38 ~Rest

Today we rest and take the day off from exercising. Keep your food intake sensibly and healthy! Have fun!!

Day 39 ~Upper Body

<u>Pre-Workout Stretch</u>

Begin your routine by stretching your legs, arms, and neck muscles. Hold each stretch for a minimum of 20-30 seconds. This includes your hamstrings, quadriceps, glutes, calves, shoulders, back, stomach, triceps, and biceps. Remember, stretching prior to working out helps prevent injury. Throughout your exercise, remember to breathe regularly. Take in deep breaths through your nose and release them out through your mouth.

<u>Cardio</u>

Treadmill

- Walk 30 minutes
- Random Mode
- 3.5 mph
- Level 5

Push-Ups

Assume a facedown position on the floor with your feet together. Place your hands on the floor, palms down; shoulder width apart. Curl your toes up toward your head. Pull your inner strength from your core and tighten your stomach and butt muscles. Raise yourself up using your arms. Allow your hands and the balls of your feet to support your weight. Make a straight line from your head to your heels. Lower your torso to the ground until your elbows form a 90 degree angle. Keep your elbows close to your body to add more resistance. Your head should be facing forward. Lower your torso as far to the ground as you can. Raise yourself up by attempting to push the ground away from you. Breathe out as you push. Continue to push yourself up until your arms are almost in a straight position. Do not lock your arms. Complete 3 sets of 6.

Front Shoulder Lift- 5lb Weights

Start this exercise standing in an upright position. Hold 5 lb. dumbbells in each hand. Let your arms hang in front of your thighs. Pull your strength from your inner core and hold your butt and stomach muscles tight.

Raise both hands straight out in front of you to shoulder height. Lower your arms back down to the starting position. Repeat. Complete 3 sets of 10.

Side Shoulder Lift-5lb Weights

Start this exercise standing in an upright position. Hold 5 lb. dumbbells in each hand. Let your arms hang down the sides of your body. Pull your strength from your inner core and hold your butt and stomach muscles tight. Ensure your elbows are slightly bent and your palms are facing inward. Raise both hands outward to the sides to shoulder height. Keep the bend in your elbows. Lower your arms back down to the starting position. Repeat. Complete 3 sets of 10.

Cool Down Stretch

End your routine by stretching your legs, arms, and neck muscles. Hold each stretch for a minimum of 20-30 seconds. This includes your hamstrings, quadriceps, glutes, calves, shoulders, back, stomach, triceps and biceps. Take deep breaths in through your nose and out through your mouth.

Day 40 - Cardio Only

<u>Pre-Workout Stretch</u>

Begin your routine by stretching your legs, arms, and neck muscles. Hold each stretch for a minimum of 20-30 seconds. This includes your hamstrings, quadriceps, glutes, calves, shoulders, back, stomach, triceps, and biceps. Remember, stretching prior to working out helps prevent injury. Throughout your exercise, remember to breathe regularly. Take in deep breaths through your nose and release them out through your mouth.

<u>Cardio</u>

Elliptical

- 30 minutes in forward direction
- At the 10, 15, and 20 minute interval marks add an "Energy Shot" by increasing your speed and pedaling faster for 30-60 seconds. Resume normal speed.
- Level 5
- 5.0 mph

<u>Cool Down Stretch</u>

End your routine by stretching your legs, arms, and neck muscles. Hold each stretch for a minimum of 20-30 seconds. This includes your hamstrings, quadriceps, glutes, calves, shoulders, back, stomach, triceps and biceps. Take deep breaths in through your nose and out through your mouth.

Day 41 -Rest

Take a break and enjoy a day of rest! You have definitely earned it! You are now about one and a half months into your new healthy lifestyle. Exercising and eating right have now become a part of your life and are becoming habits. Discipline is key! On the days you do not work out, you may begin to feel de-ja-vu because it feels like something is missing. Excellence is a habit! We are what we repeatedly do! You are on a journey of excellence so smile, be happy and live it! As always, don't forget to keep your eating healthy and sensible.

Day 42 -Lower Body

Pre-Workout Stretch

Begin your routine by stretching your legs, arms, and neck muscles. Hold each stretch for a minimum of 20-30 seconds. This includes your hamstrings, quadriceps, glutes, calves, shoulders, back, stomach, triceps, and biceps. Remember, stretching prior to working out helps prevent injury. Throughout your exercise, remember to breathe regularly. Take in deep breaths through your nose and release them out through your mouth.

Cardio

Treadmill

- Walk 30 minutes
- Random Mode
- 3.5 mph
- Level 6

Side Skips

Begin this exercise standing in an upright position. Stand with your legs spread shoulder width apart. Pull your strength from your inner core and hold your stomach and butt muscles tight. Bend your arms up towards your chin, holding your fists balled up in a fighting stance position. Keep your elbows stable and pulled in towards your sides. Start moving from side to side in a quick hopping (skipping) motion. Continue to hop (skip) for 60 seconds. Repeat 3 times.

Sumo Squats

Begin this exercise in a sitting squat stance with your feet wider than shoulder width apart. Point your toes outward and position your knees over your toes. Keep your back straight, your chest out, and hold your ab and butt muscles tight. Squat down until your thighs are parallel to the floor. Sit back into the squat keeping your weight on your heels while maintaining your posture. Slowly lift yourself back up by pushing up off your heels until you are back in the starting position. Remember your breathing when working out. Inhale on the way down and exhale on the way up. Complete this exercise slow in a controlled manner. This is not a speed exercise. Complete 3 sets of 10. (See pictures on next page).

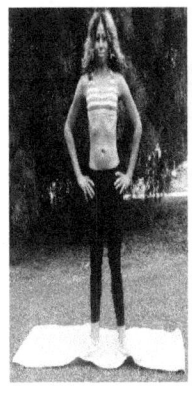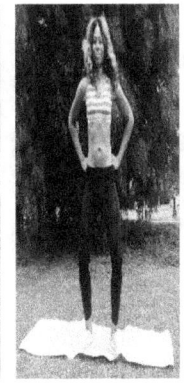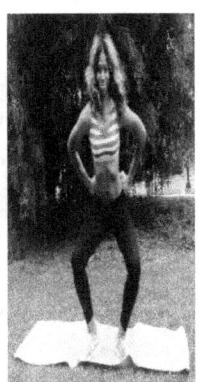

Front Skips

Begin this exercise standing in an upright position. Stand with your right leg slightly bent and about 3-4 inches ahead of your left leg. Hold your stomach and butt muscles tight. Bend your arms up toward your chin holding your fists balled up in a fighting stance position. Keep your elbows stable and pull them in towards your sides. Start moving from front to back in a quick hopping (skipping) motion. Continue to hop (skip) for 60 seconds. Repeat 3 times.

Cool Down Stretch

End your routine by stretching your legs, arms, and neck muscles. Hold each stretch for a minimum of 20-30 seconds. This includes your hamstrings, quadriceps, glutes, calves,

shoulders, back, stomach, triceps and biceps. Take deep breaths in through your nose and out through your mouth.

Chapter 9

Week 7 Days 43-49

W eek 7! This week we will continue
to maximize strength training;
however, this week we will
increase our weights to 8 lb. dumbbell
weights. We will also keep varying our
workout intensity days by adding Energy
Shots on some days of our workouts.
Measure your waistline, your left thigh and
weigh yourself. Write down the results in
your journal. Remember to breathe, keep
your water close by and have fun! Let's go!

Day 43 -Cardio Only

<u>Pre-Workout Stretch</u>

Begin your routine by stretching your legs, arms, and neck muscles. Hold each stretch for a minimum of 20-30 seconds. This includes your hamstrings, quadriceps, glutes, calves, shoulders, back, stomach, triceps, and biceps. Remember, stretching prior to working out helps prevent injury. Throughout your exercise, remember to breathe regularly. Take in deep breaths through your nose and release them out through your mouth.

<u>Cardio</u>

Elliptical

- 30 minutes in forward direction
- Level 5
- 5.1 mph

<u>Cool Down Stretch</u>

End your routine by stretching your legs, arms, and neck muscles. Hold each stretch for a minimum of 20-30 seconds. This includes your hamstrings, quadriceps, glutes, calves, shoulders, back, stomach, triceps and biceps.

Take deep breaths in through your nose and out through your mouth.

Day 44 -Upper Body

<u>Pre-Workout Stretch</u>

Begin your routine by stretching your legs, arms, and neck muscles. Hold each stretch for a minimum of 20-30 seconds. This includes your hamstrings, quadriceps, glutes, calves, shoulders, back, stomach, triceps, and biceps. Remember, stretching prior to working out helps prevent injury. Throughout your exercise, remember to breathe regularly. Take in deep breaths through your nose and release them out through your mouth.

<u>Cardio</u>

Treadmill

- Walk 30 minutes
- At the 10, 15, and 20 minute interval marks add an "Energy Shot" by increasing your speed and jogging faster for 30-60 seconds. Resume normal speed.
- Random Mode
- 3.5 mph

- Level 6

Jumping Jacks

Start out standing up straight with your feet together and your arms at your side. Bend your knees slightly and jump a few inches into the air. While in the air bring your legs out to the side about shoulder width apart. As you move your legs outward, raise your arms up over your head. Be sure your arms are slightly bent throughout the movement. Your feet should land shoulder width or wider apart as your hands meet above your head. Repeat this motion in a quick manner for 30-60 seconds. Repeat 3 times.

Bicep Curls-8 lb. Dumbbell Weights

Stand in an upright position with your feet shoulder width apart. Place your elbows against your hip bones, letting your arms slightly hang with an 8 lb. dumbbell weight in each hand. Contract your stomach ad butt muscles, holding them tight. Slowly lift both arms up together until your forearms reach your chest. Lower your arm back down to the starting position ensuring your elbows remain against your hip bones. Complete 3 sets of 12.

Shoulder Curls- 5lb. Dumbbell Weights

Stand in an upright position with your feet shoulder width apart. Hold your butt and stomach muscles tight. Hold a 5 lb. dumbbell weight in each hand. Extend both arms out to the side, keeping them level with your shoulders. Your palms should be facing up with your elbows slightly bent. Begin to curl your arms up toward your head, allowing your fists to slightly touch your shoulders. With control, begin to move your arms back outward, keeping your elbows slightly bent. Complete 3 sets of 12.

Cool Down Stretch

End your routine by stretching your legs, arms, and neck muscles. Hold each stretch for a minimum of 20-30 seconds. This includes your hamstrings, quadriceps, glutes, calves, shoulders, back, stomach, triceps and biceps. Take deep breaths in through your nose and out through your mouth.

Day 45 -Rest

Take a breather and enjoy your day off from working out. Your food intake should be healthy and sensible.

Day 46 -Abs

<u>Pre-Workout Stretch</u>

Begin your routine by stretching your legs, arms, and neck muscles. Hold each stretch for a minimum of 20-30 seconds. This includes your hamstrings, quadriceps, glutes, calves, shoulders, back, stomach, triceps, and biceps. Remember, stretching prior to working out helps prevent injury. Throughout your exercise, remember to breathe regularly. Take in deep breaths through your nose and release them out through your mouth.

<u>Cardio</u>

Elliptical

- 30 minutes in forward direction
- Level 6
- 5.2 mph

Push-Ups

Assume a facedown position on the floor with your feet together. Place your hands on the floor, palms down; shoulder width apart. Curl your toes up toward your head. Pull your inner strength from your core and tighten your stomach and butt muscles. Raise yourself up using your arms. Allow your hands and the balls of your feet to support your weight. Make a straight line from your head to your heels. Lower your torso to the ground until your elbows form a 90 degree angle. Keep your elbows close to your body to add more resistance. Your head should be facing forward. Lower your torso as far to the ground as you can. Raise yourself up by attempting to push the ground away from you. Breathe out as you push. Continue to push yourself up until your arms are almost in a straight position. Do not lock your arms. Complete 3 sets of 6.

Squat Ab Twists

Begin this exercise in the squat position with your legs about shoulder width apart. Engage your ab and butt muscles and pull them in tight. Bend your elbows and hold your arms up toward your chin. Ball your hands into a fist. Begin to twist your ab muscles from left to right in a quick motion. Continue this exercise for 30 seconds. Repeat 3 times.

Dead Lifts-8 lb. Dumbbell Weights

Start this exercise standing up in an upright position with your knees slightly bent and your legs close together. Allow your arms to hang loosely with an 8 lb. dumbbell weight in each hand. Come forward slowly bending at the waist. As you are bending over towards your legs, keep your back straight and parallel to the ground. Hold your stomach and butt muscles tight. While you are in position bending at the waist, complete a shoulder press by pulling your arms up toward your shoulders and releasing them back down. Gradually come back up to a standing position. As you reach the top, be sure to seal the exercise by giving your butt muscles a firm, tight squeeze. Complete 3 sets of 10.

Cool Down Stretch

End your routine by stretching your legs, arms, and neck muscles. Hold each stretch for a minimum of 20-30 seconds. This includes your hamstrings, quadriceps, glutes, calves,

shoulders, back, stomach, triceps and biceps. Take deep breaths in through your nose and out through your mouth.

Day 47 -Cardio Only

<u>Pre-Workout Stretch</u>

Begin your routine by stretching your legs, arms, and neck muscles. Hold each stretch for a minimum of 20-30 seconds. This includes your hamstrings, quadriceps, glutes, calves, shoulders, back, stomach, triceps, and biceps. Remember, stretching prior to working out helps prevent injury. Throughout your exercise, remember to breathe regularly. Take in deep breaths through your nose and release them out through your mouth.

<u>Cardio</u>

Treadmill

- Walk 30 minutes
- At the 10, 15, and 20 minute interval marks add an "Energy Shot" by increasing your speed and jogging faster for 30-60 seconds. Resume normal speed.
- Random Mode

- 3.5 mph
- Level 6

<u>Cool Down Stretch</u>

End your routine by stretching your legs, arms, and neck muscles. Hold each stretch for a minimum of 20-30 seconds. This includes your hamstrings, quadriceps, glutes, calves, shoulders, back, stomach, triceps and biceps. Take deep breaths in through your nose and out through your mouth.

Day 48 - Rest

You've worked hard this week! Pat yourself on the back! You've earned this day of rest. Don't forget to eat healthy and sensibly throughout the day.

Day 49 - Lower Body

<u>Pre-Workout Stretch</u>

Begin your routine by stretching your legs, arms, and neck muscles. Hold each stretch for a minimum of 20-30 seconds. This includes your hamstrings, quadriceps, glutes, calves, shoulders, back, stomach, triceps, and biceps. Remember, stretching prior to working out helps prevent injury. Throughout your exercise, remember to breathe regularly. Take in deep breaths through your nose and release them out through your mouth.

Cardio

Elliptical

- 30 minutes in forward direction
- At the 10, 15, and 20 minute intervals reverse your direction and pedal in reverse for 1 minute.
- Level 6
- 5.3 mph

Pulse Squats

Begin this exercise in a partial squat positioning your body so that you are not sitting down completely in a squat stance. Plant your feet flat on the ground about shoulder width apart. Place your hands together in front of you. Begin to pulse up and down (quick up and down movements). Continue this movement for 20-30 seconds. Repeat 3 times.

Front Kick-Back Kick

Begin this exercise standing in an upright position with your feet about hip width apart. Hold your arms up towards your chin with your fist balled in a fighting stance position. Pull your strength from your inner core and hold your butt and stomach muscles tight. Begin to lift your right leg up and kick it straight out in front of you. Place it back on the floor. Lift your left leg up and kick it back. Place it back on the floor. Complete 2 sets of 8. Switch sides, kicking your left leg front and your right leg back. Complete 2 sets of 8.

Butt Kicks

As you may recall the butt kick exercises are completed while running in place. Position your body in an upright standing form. Your feet should be about shoulder width apart. Start jogging in place. As you are jogging in place, ensure your butt and stomach muscles are engaged and tightened. While jogging, bring your heels to your glutes allowing them to touch your butt. Jog for 30-60 seconds. Repeat 3 times.

Cool Down Stretch

End your routine by stretching your legs, arms, and neck muscles. Hold each stretch for a minimum of 20-30 seconds. This includes your hamstrings, quadriceps, glutes, calves, shoulders, back, stomach, triceps and biceps. Take deep breaths in through your nose and out through your mouth.

Chapter 10

Week 8 Days 50-56

Excellence is a habit and you, my dear, are certainly there. You made the decision to change your lifestyle and get on the path to a healthier, new you! And guess what?! You did just that and are well on your way! We are now in week 8 of the healthy lifestyle change. Keep up the great work!

Day 50 - Upper Body

<u>Pre-Workout Stretch</u>

Begin your routine by stretching your legs, arms, and neck muscles. Hold each stretch for a minimum of 20-30 seconds. This includes your hamstrings, quadriceps, glutes, calves, shoulders, back, stomach, triceps, and biceps. Remember, stretching prior to working out helps prevent injury. Throughout your exercise, remember to breathe regularly. Take in deep breaths through your nose and release them out through your mouth.

<u>Cardio</u>

Treadmill

- Walk 30 minutes
- At the 10, 15, and 20 minute interval marks add an "Energy Shot" by increasing your speed and jogging faster for 30-60 seconds. Resume normal speed.
- Random Mode
- 3.6 mph
- Level 7

Front Boxer Punch with Squats

Begin this position in a squat stance. Be sure your knees are positioned behind your toes. Bend your elbows so your fists are just below your chin. Pull your strength from your inner core and hold your stomach and butt muscles tight. Punch your right arm straight out. Pull it back in. Punch your left arm straight out. Pull it back. Start moving swiftly alternating both arms. Repeat for 30-60 seconds. Complete 3 sets.

Jogging in Place-8 lb. Dumbbell Weights

Begin this exercise standing in an upright position. Place your hands at your sides holding an 8 lb. dumbbell weight in each hand. Pull your strength from your inner core and hold your ab and butt muscles tight. Begin to jog in place for 30-60 seconds. Repeat 3 times.

Reverse Plank

Begin this position sitting on the floor with your knees bent and your feet hip-width apart, flat on the floor. Place your palms on the floor on either side of your hips. Pull your strength from your inner core and hold your ab and butt muscles tight. Lift your butt off the floor until it is level with your hips and your torso is parallel to the floor. Holding this "table top" position for 30-60 seconds. Repeat 3 times.

Cool Down Stretch

End your routine by stretching your legs, arms, and neck muscles. Hold each stretch for a minimum of 20-30 seconds. This includes your hamstrings, quadriceps, glutes, calves, shoulders, back, stomach, triceps and biceps. Take deep breaths in through your nose and out through your mouth.

Day 51 -Cardio Only

Pre-Workout Stretch

Begin your routine by stretching your legs, arms, and neck muscles. Hold each stretch for a minimum of 20-30 seconds. This includes your hamstrings, quadriceps, glutes, calves, shoulders, back, stomach, triceps, and biceps. Remember, stretching prior to working out helps prevent injury. Throughout your exercise, remember to breathe regularly.

Take in deep breaths through your nose and release them out through your mouth.

<u>Cardio</u>

Elliptical

- 30 minutes in forward direction
- Level 6
- 5.4 mph

<u>Cool Down Stretch</u>

End your routine by stretching your legs, arms, and neck muscles. Hold each stretch for a minimum of 20-30 seconds. This includes your hamstrings, quadriceps, glutes, calves, shoulders, back, stomach, triceps and biceps. Take deep breaths in through your nose and out through your mouth.

<u>*Day-52-Rest*</u>

Day 52 of your healthy, lifestyle change! How fantastic is that! Take the day off and have some fun. Remember to eat healthy and sensibly throughout the day!

Day 53 - Lower Body

<u>Pre-Workout Stretch</u>

Begin your routine by stretching your legs, arms, and neck muscles. Hold each stretch for a minimum of 20-30 seconds. This includes your hamstrings, quadriceps, glutes, calves, shoulders, back, stomach, triceps, and biceps. Remember, stretching prior to working out helps prevent injury. Throughout your exercise, remember to breathe regularly. Take in deep breaths through your nose and release them out through your mouth.

<u>Cardio</u>

Treadmill

- Walk 30 minutes
- Random Mode
- 3.6 mph
- Level 7

<u>Sumo Squats</u>

Begin this exercise in a sitting squat stance with your feet wider than shoulder width apart. Point your toes outward and position your knees over your toes. Keep your back straight, your chest out, and hold your ab and butt muscles tight. Squat down until your thighs are parallel to the floor. Sit back into the squat keeping your weight on your heels while maintaining your posture. Slowly lift yourself back up by pushing up off your heels until you are back in the starting position. Remember your breathing when working out. Inhale on the way down and exhale on the way up. Complete this exercise slow in a controlled manner. This is not a speed exercise. Complete 3 sets of 10.

Skater Lunge

Begin this exercise standing in an upright position with your feet shoulder-width apart and arms at your sides. Pull your strength from your inner core and hold your ab and butt muscles tight. Move into the skater lunge position by taking a large step backwards with your right leg and cross it diagonally behind the left leg. Meanwhile, extend your left arm out to the side and swing the right arm across the hips. Hop about 2 feet to the right and come back to the beginning stance. Repeat with the other leg; that's one set. Complete 3 sets of 15.

Jump Squats

Begin this exercise standing in an upright position with your feet shoulder-width apart placing your arms at your sides. Pull your strength from your inner core and hold your ab and butt muscles tight. With control, lower your body into a squat position going only about two-thirds of the way down. Jump straight up with your arms pointed up toward the ceiling. When you land with your feet flat on the floor, repeat the squat jump. Complete 3 sets of 10.

Cool Down Stretch

End your routine by stretching your legs, arms, and neck muscles. Hold each stretch for a minimum of 20-30 seconds. This includes your hamstrings, quadriceps, glutes, calves, shoulders, back, stomach, triceps and biceps. Take deep breaths in through your nose and out through your mouth.

Day 54 -Cardio Only

Pre-Workout Stretch

Begin your routine by stretching your legs, arms, and neck muscles. Hold each stretch for a minimum of 20-30 seconds. This includes your hamstrings, quadriceps, glutes, calves, shoulders, back, stomach, triceps, and biceps. Remember, stretching prior to working out helps prevent injury. Throughout your exercise, remember to breathe regularly. Take in deep breaths through your nose and release them out through your mouth.

Cardio

Elliptical

- 30 minutes in forward direction
- Level 7
- 5.5 mph

Cool Down Stretch

End your routine by stretching your legs, arms, and neck muscles. Hold each stretch for a minimum of 20-30 seconds. This includes your hamstrings, quadriceps, glutes, calves, shoulders, back, stomach, triceps and biceps. Take deep breaths in through your nose and out through your mouth.

Day 55 - Rest

It's been an awesome week of working out. You've come to another day of well-deserved rest. Take a break, take a breather and enjoy yourself. Remember to keep your eating healthy and sensibly. Relax and have fun!

Day 56 - Abs

<u>Pre-Workout Stretch</u>

Begin your routine by stretching your legs, arms, and neck muscles. Hold each stretch for a minimum of 20-30 seconds. This includes your hamstrings, quadriceps, glutes, calves, shoulders, back, stomach, triceps, and biceps. Remember, stretching prior to working out helps prevent injury. Throughout your exercise, remember to breathe regularly. Take in deep breaths through your nose and release them out through your mouth.

<u>Cardio</u>

Treadmill

- Walk 30 minutes

- At the 10, 15, and 20 minute interval marks add an "Energy Shot" by increasing your speed and jogging faster for 30-60 seconds. Resume normal speed.
- Random Mode
- 3.6 mph
- Level 7

Sky-Reacher-5 lb. Weights

Stand with your feet hip width apart holding a 5 lb. dumbbell weight in each hand. Pull your strength from your inner core and hold your ab and butt muscles tight. Step forward with your left leg placing your weight on this leg. Lift your right leg up behind you. Bend forward slightly as you raise both arms over your head reaching up high. Hold your position for 30 seconds. Repeat 10 times, alternating legs.

Teaser

Begin this position lying on your back with your knees bent at a 90 degree angle and your feet lifted off the floor. Pull your strength from your inner core. Your arms should be lying flat on the floor with your palms facing down. Lift your arms up straight out raising them to shoulder length. Straighten your legs out at about a 45 degree angle. Your body should form a V. Hold this position for 2-30 seconds. With control, return to the starting position. Repeat 3 times. (See picture below).

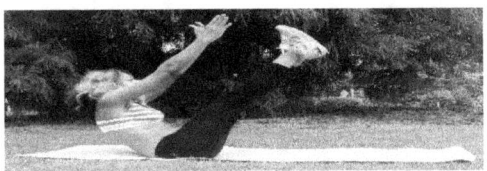

Side Plank

Start off by lying on the floor on your left side. Using your left elbow prop up the rest of your body. Position your left shoulder directly underneath your left elbow. Allow your right arm to rest on the right side of your body. Tighten your abdominal and butt muscles. Your body should be straight from your head to your feet. Do not allow your hip to sink in. Hold this position for 30-60 seconds. Complete 3 sets. Switch to your right side and complete 3 sets.

Cool Down Stretch

End your routine by stretching your legs, arms, and neck muscles. Hold each stretch for a minimum of 20-30 seconds. This includes your hamstrings, quadriceps, glutes, calves, shoulders, back, stomach, triceps and biceps.

Take deep breaths in through your nose and out through your mouth.

Chapter 11

Week 9 Days 57~60

Down to the last few days of the healthy lifestyle challenge! Track your progress by measuring your waistline, your left thigh and weigh yourself. Write down the results in your journal. Remember to breathe, keep your water close by and most importantly have fun! Let's go!

Day 57 - Cardio Only

<u>Pre-Workout Stretch</u>

Begin your routine by stretching your legs, arms, and neck muscles. Hold each stretch for a minimum of 20-30 seconds. This includes your hamstrings, quadriceps, glutes, calves, shoulders, back, stomach, triceps, and biceps. Remember, stretching prior to working out helps prevent injury. Throughout your exercise, remember to breathe regularly. Take in deep breaths through your nose and release them out through your mouth.

<u>Cardio</u>

Elliptical

- 30 minutes in forward direction
- At the 10, 15, and 20 minute interval marks add an "Energy Shot" by increasing your speed and pedaling faster for 30-60 seconds. Resume normal speed.
- Level 7
- 5.5 mph

<u>Cool Down Stretch</u>

End your routine by stretching your legs, arms, and neck muscles. Hold each stretch for a minimum of 20-30 seconds. This includes your hamstrings, quadriceps, glutes, calves, shoulders, back, stomach, triceps and biceps. Take deep breaths in through your nose and out through your mouth.

Day 58 - Lower Body

<u>Pre-Workout Stretch</u>

Begin your routine by stretching your legs, arms, and neck muscles. Hold each stretch for a minimum of 20-30 seconds. This includes your hamstrings, quadriceps, glutes, calves, shoulders, back, stomach, triceps, and biceps. Remember, stretching prior to working out helps prevent injury. Throughout your exercise, remember to breathe regularly. Take in deep breaths through your nose and release them out through your mouth.

<u>Cardio</u>

Treadmill

- Walk 30 minutes
- Random Mode
- 3.6 mph
- Level 7

Leg Circles

Begin this exercise lying on your back with your arms by your sides and your palms facing down. Pull your strength from your inner core and hold your stomach and butt muscles tight. With control, pull your right leg up towards the ceiling. Point your toes. Begin to move your whole leg in a circular motion. Keep your hip planted on the floor. Complete 5 circles in a clockwise direction. Then complete 5 circles in a counter-clockwise direction. Switch legs and repeat.

Squat with Leg Lift

Begin this exercise by standing in an upright position. Place your hands on your hips. Pull your strength from your inner core and hold your stomach and butt muscles tight. Bend your knees and lower your body into a squat position. Stand back up and lift your right leg out to the side. Bend your knees and lower your body into a squat position again. Stand up and lift your left leg out to the side Complete 3 sets of 10.

Front Knee Leg Lifts

While balancing on one leg bring the opposite leg up towards your chest slowly.

Extend your arms straight out to the sides of you. As you bring your leg up, be sure to hold it at a 90 degree angle. Pull your strength from your inner core and hold your stomach and butt muscles tight. Hold your leg up in the 90 degree angle for 10 seconds. Complete 3 sets of 10. Repeat with the other leg.

Cool Down Stretch

End your routine by stretching your legs, arms, and neck muscles. Hold each stretch for a minimum of 20-30 seconds. This includes your hamstrings, quadriceps, glutes, calves, shoulders, back, stomach, triceps and biceps. Take deep breaths in through your nose and out through your mouth.

Day 59 ~Rest

Wow! Don't you feel fantastic! Working out is a great way to clear your mind and just feel free! You've worked hard this week and earned this day off. Take today to pamper yourself but as always keep your food intake sensible and healthy.

Day 60 -Cardio Only

<u>Pre-Workout Stretch</u>

Begin your routine by stretching your legs, arms, and neck muscles. Hold each stretch for a minimum of 20-30 seconds. This includes your hamstrings, quadriceps, glutes, calves, shoulders, back, stomach, triceps, and biceps. Remember, stretching prior to working out helps prevent injury. Throughout your exercise, remember to breathe regularly. Take in deep breaths through your nose and release them out through your mouth.

Elliptical

- 20 minutes in forward direction
- 10 minutes in reverse direction
- Level 7
- 5.5 mph

<u>Cool Down Stretch</u>

End your routine by stretching your legs, arms, and neck muscles. Hold each stretch for a minimum of 20-30 seconds. This includes your hamstrings, quadriceps, glutes, calves, shoulders, back, stomach, triceps and biceps.

Take deep breaths in through your nose and out through your mouth.

Conclusion

Well ladies, our 60 day healthy lifestyle challenge has come to an end. But this is just the beginning of your healthy lifestyle. I hope that I have been able to inspire you and that you are off to a great start on your voyage of lifestyle changes. It's a wonderful feeling to be healthy. Exercising is therapeutic. I enjoy it and hope that it will find a place to stay in your heart too.

Remember all the tips and tricks you have learned over the past 60 days. Make your workout fun; enjoy yourself. Keep your water close by. Breathe! To keep your heart healthy, be sure to get at least 30 minutes of consistent cardio. To prevent a workout plateau, remember to modify your routine. Don't do the same exact workout day in and day out. Experiment with weights, keep altering your workouts and adding in your *"Energy Shots"* so that your workout routine consists of low intensity days and high intensity days. Don't forget to stretch before and after your workouts. While working out, if you need to take a break, take one…but don't give up and quit. Get right back into your routine.

Switch up your routine at times! For your cardio, take a brisk walk or jog outside on warmer days. Go for a hike. Make it a family event! My son loves going hiking with me. It's our thing. Lol. Go swimming with the kiddos. Play soccer, kickball or softball with them. Be creative. For strengthening, try rock-climbing! Ride a bike, go skating or rollerblading. Play a game of tennis. If you're near a beach, try some beach volleyball!

Before grabbing a bite to eat, ask yourself, "Am I really hungry or do I just want to eat something?" I've always liked to say we eat to live not live to eat. Remember this and it will take you far in your healthy lifestyle journey. Fad diets change your weight but working out changes your body! Good luck and I wish you much success on your continued journey to a healthy lifestyle. Always remember with God, all things are possible because He gives us strength. Stay blessed!

The End

Thank you for taking the time to read "The Everyday Mom's Guide to Being Fit & Fabulous". If you enjoyed it, please consider telling your friends or posting a short review. Word of mouth is an author's best friend and much appreciated.